RADIOGRAPHY:
Technology, Environment, Professionalism

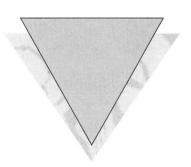

RADIOGRAPHY:
Technology, Environment, Professionalism

Frances E. Campeau, MA, RT(R)(M), FAERS

Professor and Director
Radiologic Technology Program
School of Allied Health Sciences
University of Louisville
Louisville, Kentucky

WITH THREE CONTRIBUTORS

Lippincott Williams & Wilkins

Philadelphia ● New York ● Baltimore

Acquisitions Editor: Lawrence McGrew
Editorial Assistant: Holly Chapman
Production Editor: Virginia Barishek
Production Manager: Helen Ewan
Production Service and Composition: Pine Tree Composition
Printer/Binder: R. R. Donnelley & Sons/Crawfordsville
Cover Designer: Deborah Lynam
Cover Printer: Lehigh Press

9 8 7 6 5 4 3 2 1

Library of Congress Cataloging-in-Publication Data
Campeau, Frances
    Radiography : technology, environment, professionalism / Frances
E. Campeau ; with three contributors.
       p.   cm.
    Includes bibliographical references and index.
    ISBN 0-397-55196-7
    1. Radiography, Medical—Practice. 2. Radiologic technologists.
I. Title.
    [DNLM: 1. Radiography. WN 200 C193r 1999]
RC78.C333 1999
616.07'572—dc21
DNLM/DLC
for Library of Congress   98-24217
                                                        CIP

This book is dedicated to my wonderful mother and father, who instilled in their children, Helen, Ann, David, and myself, the understanding of human respect and above all the understanding of love.

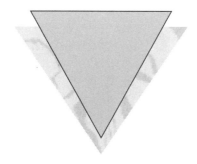

Contributors

Ellis W. Blanton, Med RT(R)(N)
Director, Radiology
Baptist Hospital East
Louisville, Kentucky
Chapter 4: The Evolution of the Hospital Radiology Department

Michael R. Bloyd, RT, RN
Director of Education Services
Tailor County Hospital
Campbellsville, Kentucky
Chapter 7: Principles of Patient Care for Imaging Technologies

A. Michael Connor, PhD
Assistant Professor
Department of Diagnostic Radiology
University of Louisville Hospital
Louisville, Kentucky
Chapter 5: Radiation Protection

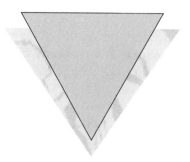

Preface

Radiography: Technology, Environment, Professionalism is unlike other books used for an introduction to the profession of radiologic technology. It looks at radiography as a high-technology discipline, a profession that combines art with science, and a patient-contact-oriented helping profession. It seeks to give the student an enhanced understanding of and reasoned respect for the profession of radiography and the radiographer.

Chapters 1 through 4 and Chapters 8 and 9 are interconnected. Chapter 8, the pivotal chapter of the book, discusses in depth the radiology environment, environmental ethics, and the radiographer's opportunities for control (independence and responsibility). Chapters 1 through 4 and 9 are intended to support and reinforce Chapter 8. Chapters 5 through 7 are overviews of technical concepts that reflect on issues discussed in the other chapters. The technical chapters are intended only as overviews of the relevant content, and it is expected that students will be provided with more detailed information in appropriately related courses as they progress through the radiography curriculum.

This book has drawn reference material from literature covering a fairly wide scope in time. The author believes that thoughts and ideas do not lose their force simply because 20 years have passed since they were set down in print; some of humanity's greatest creative ideas are hundreds and thousands of years old. Additionally, the health care delivery system is in a constant state of flux. As this book goes to print, the pendulum of interest has swung very far in the direct of cost-containment—so far, in fact, that it will almost certainly swing back towards the patient and quality-of-care issues.

There is a final consideration the author has kept in mind in preparing this book. Radiographers, or radiologic technologists, will continue to create images through a process using ionizing radiation. However, the equipment used to make images is rapidly undergoing change. It may be that in 10 years film will be the old way of doing things and almost obsolete. One does not have to be clairvoyant to see digitized imaging already replacing traditional methods and materials and becoming the state-of-the-art technique in the future. The new technologies offer advantages in patient care areas that will drive change, whether or not it is desired by current practitioners in the radiological sciences. This book has been written with the idea of helping novice radiographers and students establish a solid identity and understanding of their professional role regardless of what changes may occur in the technology they will use as practitioners.

Frances E. Campeau, MA, RT(R)(M), FAERS

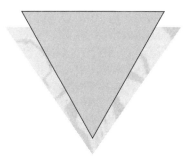

Foreword

From 1958 to 1978, I worked as a radiographer in a large, urban general hospital, where I started my career as a student. In 1978, I was serving as technical director of the department of radiology and as program director and instructor in the hospital's radiologic technology program when the program, along with several other hospital-based programs, was transferred to a local, state-supported university. The radiologic technology program moved to a newly created allied health academic unit in an emerging health sciences center; I moved from the hospital world to the world of academe. Since that time I have continued to serve as program director and faculty in the program and have climbed the academic rungs to gain a full professorship.

During the years I was a student, then a practicing radiographer and teacher in a hospital-based program, I was very aware of areas in which I had personal responsibility as well as areas in which I could exercise independence. I had a very firm idea about who I was and where I fit into the general scheme of the hospital world. As the university years have passed, I have become increasingly concerned about whether students learning to become radiographers in the academic milieu develop the same sense of worth and awareness of their professional role which were the natural outcomes of attending hospital-based programs. There are, of course, many advantages to obtaining an education and degree in a postsecondary institution; the educational and cultural bases are necessarily broader and the graduate has more options for practice and to pursue further educational goals. However, the hospital is, comparatively, a little pond and the university a big one. Although students still spend many hours in clinical, they are not there as insiders in the same way that the student radiographer was in a hospital-based program. Personally, I believe both educational settings offer advantages and disadvantages.

The idea for *Radiography: Technology, Environment, Professionalism* has been with me for a long time. Around 1980 I began to think that education of the radiographer should include some new themes, or elaboration on existing themes, that would make the professional role of the radiographer more distinct and meaningful to the student. I especially wanted to help students recognize their opportunities for independence as practitioners and also to recognize their responsibility for their own work. However, I felt that writing this particular book would be a true challenge because parts of it might question patterns of thinking which have become comfortable for many of us.

When I decided to start the book, I invited my friend and colleague, Nancy C. Roubieu, a member of the administrative staff in allied health, to work with me as the book's primary editor. For the past seventeen years she has provided this type of staff support to various faculty members in both allied health and nursing. Additionally, we had worked together on a number of projects previously—research papers, a self-learning study manual for the state, another published book, reaccreditation self-studies, and the like. Over the years she has developed an unusual introductory knowledge base in many areas in allied health and nursing—I knew she would be able to make contributions to this book that would be very useful. In fact, she suggested using the radiographers' code of ethics to define the elements of a professional role for radiographers. Nancy also has the knack of knowing what I mean when I occasionally struggle to express myself and helps me reframe my words so the meaning is clear. She agreed to work on the book with me, we prepared a prospectus, and it was accepted. Had either of us known what obstacles (illness, accidents, tragedy) would lie in our way as we worked on this book, most likely we would never have started. In any event, without Nancy's collaboration, contributions, and editing, this particular book would not have become a reality. I am indebted to her for seeing this project through and want to recognize her ongoing support and contributions to the school and its faculty.

I want to acknowledge several other persons who have contributed to the book in different ways: my program assistant, Deborah S. Kaufmann, for helping me in a thousand different ways; my colleagues and fellow faculty members, Ann M. Obergfell and Don A. Pack, for their support and forbearance; Kay Lloyd and Gerald Johnson of the University of Louisville Hospital for their rapid response to my requests for information regarding hospital policies and accreditation; and my good friend, Carol L. Cornette, for providing art work for Chapters 2 and 8. I am also extremely grateful to the contributing authors who wrote chapters for the book: Ellis Blanton (Chapter 4), Dr. Michael Connor (Chapter 5), and Michael Bloyd (Chapter 7).

There is one other person I would like to acknowledge and that is Nettie G. King, M.D., the medical director of the University of Louisville Radiologic Technology Program. As a medical professional, Dr. King's participation and instruction in the program validate the essence of this book, in both her respect for radiographers and the high expectation she holds for the profession. Dr. King reflects the collegial relationship between physicians and radiographers that ideally should prevail in all radiology environments—hospitals, offices, clinics, or mobile units. She is teacher, guide, and advocate.

Frances E. Campeau, MA, RT(R)(M), FAERS

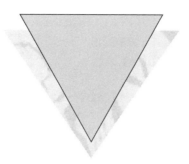

Contents

II Introduction to the Practice of Radiography 83

5 RADIATION PROTECTION **85**

6 OVERVIEW OF RADIOGRAPHIC EXPOSURES **103**

RADIOGRAPHY:
Technology, Environment, Professionalism

UNIT

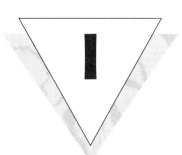

I

Introduction to the Profession of Radiography

CHAPTER

The Radiographer

3

▶ OBJECTIVES

At the conclusion of the learning opportunity the reader will be able to:

1. Explain why the first "technicians" or assistants were used by radiologists.
2. List the elements of the radiographer's professional role.
3. Note some similarities and differences between the professions of radiologist and radiologic technologist.
4. Give a thumbnail sketch of the development of radiography as a profession.
5. List and briefly describe various imaging modalities.
6. Explain why the way people perceive themselves may be affected by how they are perceived by others.

▶ EVOLUTION OF THE PROFESSIONAL ROLE

The story of radiology in the twentieth century has been one of rapidly changing and ever-expanding technology, one that has kept radiologists and their companion professionals on the cutting edge of advances in medicine and the development of the radiological sciences. Within this century, the knowledge base for the practice of medical radiology, as well as for related radiation sciences (e.g., radiation physics, radiation biology), has undergone continual growth. Particularly in the second half of the century, since the end of World War II heralded the arrival of atomic energy, whole bodies of knowledge have evolved related to the effects of radiation on the human body, safe use of radiation, and the dangers of prolonged radiation exposure.

The profession of radiographer evolved as physicians practicing the emerging discipline of radiology found they needed assistance in the actual recording of images—that "picture taking" was a time-consuming practice and one quite different from reading radiographs for medical diagnostic purposes or planning therapeutic regimens.

Although the profession of radiographer developed in tandem with that of the diagnostic radiologist, the two professional roles necessarily differ. A radiologist is a physician and shares elements of that professional role with all other physicians, whether in the same or other medical disciplines. The role of physician is well recognized and held in high regard by other members of the health care team and by the general public. The professional role of the radiographer is understood less well by the public and is often undervalued even within the discipline itself.

Elements of the radiographer's professional role—technically competent practitioner, ethically competent practitioner, advocate for radiation safety and protection, patient care services provider, and user of initiative and independent judgment in applying radiologic techniques—have not been identified and advanced in the same way or as vigorously as some other health professions have defined and promulgated functions of their roles. For example, similar to nurses, radiographers have "hands-on" patient contact and must be prepared to provide routine patient care and to handle patient care emergencies in addition to performing the nuts-and-bolts tasks of radiography. Yet, the general public often does not know or understand that the radiographer's role includes some critical aspects of the nurse's role with respect to direct patient care.

Because radiographers often perform as nameless members of the health care team in media representations as well as in real life, it is not surprising that the general public is not well informed about the radiographer's role. It is important, however, that radiographers understand their role and that it is critical to health care. The key point here, then, is for beginning radiographers to realize they are being prepared to fill a professional role and to begin to relate what they are learning in the academic and clinical settings to different facets of that role.

Another aspect of the radiographer's role is worth noting. Early in the practice of radiology, "most radiographers were photographers or physicians who practiced photography as a hobby" [6, p. 6]. The terms often used today in learning the mechanics of radiography—that is, light, films, filters, screens, developing solutions, drying, and so on—are universal terms that also apply to photography. Although most of us pick up a camera now and then and take snapshots, few actually have studied photographic composition, have more than a button-pushing understanding of cameras, or know how to develop film and print pictures. Those persons who master the medium and pursue photography at a professional level are generally regarded as a type of artist. Radiographers should not lose sight of the relationship of radiography to photography—that as radiographers, they are, in a sense, artists.

▶ BRIEF HISTORY

Viewed from a wide perspective, Wilhem Conrad Röntgen's discovery of x-radiation on November 8, 1895, although accidental to his research intent, can be seen as one of many breakthroughs in mankind's search to understand and control the forces and elements affecting human health and well-being. We can catch a glimpse of primitive man's beliefs and practices in the evidence of prehistoric remains found scattered here and there around the world and also from the study of primitive societies still in existence today. In such societies, diagnosis was (and is) very often associated with magic or with divination rites. The witch doctor, shaman, medicine man, or primitive priest usually followed prescribed ceremonies to uncover and drive out the source of an illness, although illness was often ascribed to demons or spirits rather than to physical causes. In uncovering or determining the source of illness, these priests/magicians acted as primitive diagnosticians.

The evolution of medical diagnosis extends from primitive man to the technology of today. It is important for the radiographer to realize that the practice of medical diagnosis is both as new as today's technology and as old as mankind.

Radiology

Although Röntgen's discovery is extremely important, a number of historical purists might contend that radiology can trace its history to the year 1600 when Gilbert "created the foundation for the sciences of magnetism and electricity" [5, p. 1]. Although no one will deny that the discovery of x-rays is the foundation upon which radiology is built, there is little doubt that many others contributed to its development and growth. For instance, Röntgen was working with a Crookes-Hittorf tube when he made his discovery. The work of many others helped lay the scientific foundation for the advent of radiology. Table 1-1 is a chronological list (not inclusive) of scientists and their discoveries or theories from 1600 to 1893.

Following Röntgen's breakthrough, many scientists, physicians, and others, recognizing the importance of this phenomenal ray, began working in experimentation and research with x-rays. Developments, discoveries, and improvements in the field took place rapidly in the next 100 years. As early as 1898, Edison developed the first fluoroscope; many individuals—Becquerel, Rutherford, the

TABLE 1-1

List of Scientists and Their Discoveries/Theories, 1600 to 1893

Year	Scientist	Area of Work/Discovery
1600	Gilbert	Created the foundation for the sciences of magnetism and electricity.
1675	Newton	Built a more efficient electrostatic generator with a rotating glass sphere.
1729	Gray	Distinguished conductors of electricity from non-conductors.
1733	du Fay	Discovered two different types of electricity, vitreous and resinous electricity.
1747	Watson	Transmitted electricity over long conductors.
1750	Franklin	Defined positive and negative electricity.
1786	Galvani	Discovered animal electricity.
1800	Volta	Constructed the first electrical battery, the Voltaic pile.
1820	Oersted	Discovered the link between electricity and magnetism.
1820	Ampere	Formulated mathematically the discovery of Oersted.
1827	Ohm	Formulated Ohm's laws, stating the relations between electric current, electromotive force, and resistance.
1831	Faraday and Henry	Discovered electromagnetic induction.
1836	Sturgeon and Page	Built the first induction coil.
1850	Plucker	Observed green-glass fluorescence opposite the negative electrode in a vacuum tube.
1858	Kohlrausch and Lord Kelvin	Improved electrometers.
1860	Toepler, Holtz, and Wimshurst	Improved electrostatic machines.
1860	Geissler	Developed vacuum tubes containing various gases and found that some bases become luminous when high-tension discharges are passed through the tube.
1869	Hittorf	Observed many of the properties of cathode rays.
1873	Maxwell	Published his famous equations in the book, *Treatise on Electricity and Magnetism.*
1879	Crookes	Found that cathode rays can be deflected by a magnet and believed that he was dealing with "fourth state of matter."
1885	Hertz	Proved Maxwell's equations by experimental methods.

Note: Adapted from *Physical Foundations of Radiology* (3rd ed., pp. 1–3), by O. Glass, E. H. Quimby, L. S. Taylor, J. L. Weatherwax, and R. H. Morgan, 1965, New York: Harper & Row, Publishers, Incorporated.

Curies, Planck, Soddy, Compton, Eastman, Coolidge, Snook, Lawrence, to name a few—contributed to continuing advancements in radiology.

Radiography

Perhaps one of the most important things about their own history for radiographers to keep in mind is that *radiologists*, or röntgenologists, had to struggle to establish their discipline as a branch of medicine. Initially, they were held in relatively low opinion among other specialists but were able to correct this unsatisfactory perception and become recognized as physicians equal to other physician specialists.

The history of radiography also includes a struggle for recognition, including recognition from radiologists as well as from other health providers and the general public. Eddy Clifford Jerman was the first strong proponent for defining the role of the technicians who took radiographs and for establishing an information base for educating them in technique.

Jerman's education, work experience, and life experience virtually predestined him to become a person of consequence in the developing field of radiographic equipment and x-ray production. By adding a Crookes tube to already existing equipment, he began experimenting in the field in March 1896 [6]. Thereafter, he worked as an x-ray equipment manufacturer, salesman, installer, repairer, demonstrator, and lecturer for a number of years with varying degrees of financial success and failure.

In 1916, at a point where he was distressed financially and suffering guilt feelings about how his lack of success was affecting his family, he began sorting out the pieces of information he had gained through nearly twenty years of experience in the field [6]. Subsequently, he proposed that "all men interested in x-ray work—the manufacturer, the salesman, the technician, and the doctor should be intensely interested in the end results, the bringing about of the best possible result for the patient. . . . Three great essentials are involved in the success or failure of any x-ray laboratory—equipment, technique and interpretation" [6, p. 34]. Jerman then decided that instruction in technique was the single most critical problem in x-ray production—the "weakest link of the chain"—and that he would "devote the rest of my life work in an effort toward strengthening this link" [6, p. 34]. After an inauspicious beginning (it was difficult to locate a doctor willing to pay for instruction in equipment usage), Jerman began to experience the success he had so long sought and the realization of his vision. "On May 20, 1917, Victor [the x-ray company with whom Jerman most wanted to affiliate] established its Educational Department with Jerman as its head" [6, p. 35].

Formal education in radiographic techniques largely evolved from the foundation laid by Jerman. Additionally, he helped initiate the development of the professional organizations that would represent practitioners, author their code of ethics, and help establish guidelines and maintain standards for education in and the practice of radiography. With Jerman as the initiator, efforts to organize began in October 1920. He pointed the effort in the direction of a true professional organization, although labor unions were commonly popular at the time and that kind of association was favored by many technicians [6]. The organization was named the American Association of Radiological Technicians (AART) at the first meeting, met again in 1922, but did not hold another meeting until 1926. During the interim, radiologists became involved in formally establishing the technician's role in the practice of radiology.

In the early 1920s organized radiology, through its own professional organizations, "decided that some form of recognition of x-ray technicians should be established . . . (and) that a technician Registry be established to certify technicians meeting certain qualifications" [6, p. 41]. Radiologists, having struggled to gain credibility for themselves, understood the need for technicians to establish an identity and gain recognition for their professional role. Thus, they were tentatively supportive of the technicians' desire to organize professionally, as long as that organization did not involve unionization. However, radiologists were somewhat fearful that technicians, registered or not, might strive for independence through establishing lay laboratories; in other words, they might compete with radiologists. Additionally, because radiologists were most often men and the vast majority of technicians were women, "the job loyalties of the day demanded that the female employee obey his orders" [6, pp. 42–43]; attempts to organize might have been perceived as an unwelcome show of assertiveness on the part of women.

Through the efforts of two professional radiologist societies, the American Roentgen Ray Society and the Radiological Society of North America, the American Registry of Radiological Technicians was developed and "officially came into being early in 1923" [6, p. 43]. Thus, basic application standards for x-ray production and the first certifying examinations for technicians were in place within thirty years of Röntgen's discovery. Additionally, efforts to organize x-ray technicians professionally were underway only twenty years after similar activity by the radiologists. Table 1-2 lists significant dates and events in the evolution of radiography as a profession.

Two additional points are worth remembering in terms of the evolution of the early radiologic sciences disciplines. The first relates to the fact that strong linkages were forged between the technicians and the manufacturers of equipment and photographic supplies and their representatives. This relationship provided both tangible and intangible assistance to the development of educational programs and guidelines and standards for equipment usage. This relationship still exists today to a degree unusual in the current health-care delivery system. Secondly, it should be noted that radiation therapy developed almost in parallel with radiography and that therapeutic applications of nuclear medicine had been applied experimentally in the 1930s. Equipment for using nuclear medicine as a diagnostic tool was being manufactured by the late 1940s, with significant technological advances appearing steadily thereafter. Thus, radiography, radiation therapy, and nuclear medicine share elements of a common history in the development of the radiologic sciences.

Much has happened in radiography during the years from the early 1920s to the late 1990s. Standards for training and education have continued to be developed and augmented; as a result of safety issues that became apparent from exposure to radiation, standards for radiation protection have been established; bodies of knowledge related to radiation physics and radiation biology have emerged and relevant information is included in radiographer education; the title *technician* was changed to *technologist* in the 1960s (the earlier term was seen as being limited since the advent of new radiologic sciences technologies and disciplines appeared); attitude changes about educational standards in the late 1960s and early 1970s created a climate in which radiography education started moving from hospital-based training programs to academia; and changes in the health-care delivery system and health-care financing have made it desirable for technologists to become multicompetent in various imaging modalities. These various modalities will be defined and discussed in the next section of this chapter.

TABLE 1-2

Events and Evolution of Organizations Related to Professional Radiologic Technology*

Year	Event
1920	Thirteen technicians, along with radiologists and x-ray manufacturer representatives, were brought together by Jerman for a meeting that resulted in formation of a new association, the American Association of Radiological Technicians (AART), and adoption of a constitution and bylaws (pp. 38–39).
1921	The first annual meeting of the AART was held in Chicago.
1923	The American Registry of Radiological Technicians (ARRT), created as a certifying body largely at the mandate of radiologist organizations, was officially recognized, although certification had begun in November 1922 (p. 43).
1925	"Officers of the AART and the Registry met and agreed to restrict membership in the national professional association to registered technicians" (p. 45).
1926	A reorganization meeting of the AART was held at which changes were made in the bylaws that discontinued associate memberships (and thus eliminated non-technicians).
1926	Organization of regional societies, which began in 1922, expanded.
1927	A survey of radiologists was conducted by the Registry to determine if they still supported the organization; a majority of the radiologists favored continuing the Registry (p. 46).
1929	The first issue of the journal of the AART, *The X-Ray Technician*, was published.
1930	The name of the AART organization was changed to American Society of Radiographers (ASR); the ASR was given representation on the Registry Board.
1931	An annual meeting (6th) was held at a site other than Chicago.
1931	"A Council on Education and Registration was created in cooperation with the Radiological Society of North America" (RSNA) with the charge to work toward establishing a curriculum "for radiographers in educational institutions" (p. 54).
1933	The RSNA Council on Education Registration recommendations were adopted; recommendations addressed areas related to candidates' age, health, and personality; site of educational program; minimum duration of the course; and subjects to be included in the course of instruction.
1934	The name of the ASR was officially changed to American Society of X-Ray Technicians (ASXT).
1936	The ARRT changed its name to the American Registry of X-Ray Technicians (ARXT).
1937	The "International X-Ray and Radiation Protection Commission issued new safety guidelines for full-time x-ray workers" (p. 62).
1939	The ASXT adopted a resolution declaring itself against unionism (p. 62).

TABLE 1-2 *Continued*

Year	Event
1943–1945	Annual meetings of the ASXT were suspended because of the war effort and governmental restrictions on transportation; however, state societies continued to meet.
1943	The American College of Radiology (ACR) replaced the RSNA as co-sponsor of the Registry with the ASXT (p. 72).
1944	The American Medical Association's Council on Medical Education and Hospitals assumed responsibility for approving schools for x-ray technicians (p. 73).
1952	The Education Committee of the ASXT submitted a model standardized curriculum for x-ray technician education to the ACR for approval; the curriculum was approved later in the year (p. 87).
1955	The ASXT created a membership category known as Fellow to recognize leaders of the profession.
1963	A change in the Registry's name to the American Registry of Radiologic Technologists (ARRT) was implemented.
1963	The first "isotope" (nuclear medicine) certifying examination was administered (p. 110).
1964	The ASXT changed its name to the American Society of Radiologic Technologists (ASRT).
1964	"The first radiation therapist certification examination was administered" (p. 110).
1966	"The Registry began restricting certification [of technologists] to graduates of AMA-approved programs" (p. 116).
1969	The Joint Review Committee on Educational Programs in Radiologic Technology was formed by the ASRT and the ACR (p. 122).
1979	"The ASRT petitioned the National Labor Relations Board [NLRB] to change the radiologic technologist's status from 'technical' to professional" (p. 123). The NLRB did not agree to a general rule change.
1980	The ACR "adopted a statement recognizing radiologic technologists as 'professional members of the health care team'" (p. 123).
1981	"The Consumer-Patient Radiation Health and Safety Act . . . was passed by both houses of Congress. . . . The act required the Secretary of Health and Human Services to develop federal standards for the certification of radiologic technologists and the accreditation of educational programs in radiologic technology . . . [and] to provide the states with a model statute for licensure. Compliance by states was voluntary" (p. 125).
1991	The first cardiovascular-interventional technology certifying examination was administered.
1992	The first mammography certifying examination was administered.
1995	The first certifying examinations for computed tomography and magnetic resonance imaging were administered.
1997	The first certifying examination quality management was administered.

*Most data selected or excerpted from *The Shadowmakers* by E. L. Harris, 1995, Albuquerque: American Society of Radiologist Technologists. Direct quotes are identified by page number.

▶ VARIOUS IMAGING MODALITIES

Imaging modalities available today in the practice of radiology reflect the rapid pace of technical advancement during the past century. In the following discussion, we will briefly examine modalities, or services, offered in the modern hospital radiology department. Although radiographers practice in other environments, the hospital is the establishment where the fullest range of imaging modalities is most likely to be present.

X-ray

In 1993 Bushong pointed out that there are two general types of x-ray procedures: (1) radiographic examinations producing fixed photographic images and (2) fluoroscopic examinations producing dynamic images revealed through fluoroscopy [2]. Although this principle of image production in x-ray has not changed a great deal, there have been many improvements since x-rays became a common diagnostic tool. For example, today the x-ray generator is computer controlled for increased precision in setting techniques for radiographs and fluoroscopic images. Additionally, currently "many areas of x-ray diagnosis require special equipment and techniques to obtain diagnostic information . . . (such areas) include tomography, stereoradiography, and magnification radiography" [3, p. 262].

Vascular and Interventional Radiography

Retrograde arteriography procedures are performed by the radiologist or other qualified physician. This procedure is done under fluoroscopic guidance by insertion of a guide wire into the femoral artery followed by a catheter that moves along the guide wire to the area of interest. Contrast is injected by a pressure or power injector. In some rare instances the brachial artery may be the approach used for these procedures.

Interventional techniques are also commonly used. Angioplasty, thrombolysis, stents, and grafts are being performed to resolve clots, occlusions, and stenosis. Procedures called embolotherapy are being done to occlude arteries supplying blood to tumors or an arteriovenous malformation.

Nuclear Medicine

Nuclear medicine, although it is also an imaging modality, is quite different from radiography. It is the "branch of radiology that uses *radionuclides* [radioisotopes]—unstable atoms that emit radiation spontaneously—in the diagnosis and treatment of disease" [8, p. 11]. The modern camera can perform planar imaging to cover the entire body as well as tomographic imaging.

The computer has had a dramatic impact on nuclear medicine as it has in all other areas of radiology. In today's nuclear medicine laboratory, almost all imaging procedures are obtained or manipulated with the use of computer applications. Single photon emission tomography (SPECT) utilizes a computer technique coupled with a transverse section imaging device to produce transaxial tomograms of the body [4].

An emergent technology is positron emission imaging, or PET, which uses extremely short-lived nuclides to image the brain to obtain information related to dementia, psychosis, and epilepsy. In some nuclear medicine labs, monoclonal antibody labeling is being done and used in some imaging procedures. This technique opens the door to not only diagnostic imaging but to possibilities for localized therapeutic procedures as well.

Ultrasound

Ultrasonography is a modality that requires special equipment and is used to "produce an image or photograph of an organ or tissue. Ultrasonic echoes are recorded as they strike tissues of different densities" [9, p. 2069]. Ultrasound is an "inaudible sound in the frequency range of approximately 20,000 to 10 billion (10^9) cycles per second. Ultrasound has different velocities in tissues that differ in density and elasticity from others. This property permits the use of ultrasound in outlining the shape of various tissues and organs" [9, p. 2069].

General ultrasound procedures are used in pelvic, abdominal, obstetrical and gynecological, and pediatric imaging. Ultrasound plays a major role in obstetrics and in the diagnosis of gynecologic disorders. Abdominal ultrasound procedures continue to increase as a result of today's technology and the economics of managed care. For diagnosis of right upper quadrant pain or pelvic pain, ultrasound is an excellent place to start. The procedure is cost-effective, easy to do, accessible and quick, and may give the answer to the problem.

Ultrasound has also become an important adjunct to mammography when an attempt is made to confirm a cyst or a solid lesion. Ultrasound is also used to guide core biopsies. There is general consensus that there will be increased biopsy procedures done under ultrasound guidance because, again, it is easier and more economical to do than surgical procedures.

Echocardiography is "a noninvasive diagnostic method that uses ultrasound . . . to visualize internal cardiac structures. All cardiac valves can be visualized and the dimensions of each ventricle and the left atrium can be measured" [9, p. 601]. Ultrasound methods are potentially useful in the diagnosis of abnormalities of other organs as well.

Mammography

Simply stated, mammography is "radiography of the soft tissues of the breast to allow identification of various benign and malignant neoplastic processes" [1, p. 636]. This area of medical imaging has become something of a specialty within most radiology departments and has been an area of great public interest for the past several years as a screening method for early detection of breast cancer. There is still disagreement in the medical profession over the age women should begin having routine (every two years of every year) mammograms.

Although procedures for imaging the breast have been performed since the 1920s, available techniques did not produce quality radiographs and initially required high dosages of radiation. In the 1970s and 1980s as low-dose film screen techniques were introduced, they became the techniques of choice for mammography. Subsequently, the procedure gained wide acceptance as a highly regarded early detection screening tool.

CT Scanning

Computer tomography (CT) is "an x-ray technique that produces a film representing a detailed cross section of tissue structure. The procedure uses a . . . (fan-shaped) beam of x-rays that rotates in a . . . 360-degree motion around the patient to image the body in cross-sectional slices. An array of detectors . . . records those x-rays that pass through the body. The image is created by computer" [1, p. 250]. Many persons involved in radiology believe this modality revolutionized the practice of radiology. Certainly, compared to conventional x-rays, CT scanning has dramatically increased the diagnostic information that can be obtained through imaging [7].

Over the years, CT scanners have continually shown improvement. Today, several techniques have been developed that add information to the basic CT cross-sectional image. All CT scanners can produce an image projection radiograph comparable to a plain film radiograph. Dynamic imaging, a technique useful in imaging to obtain vascularity of lesions or structures, produces rapid, repetitive image acquisitions without reconstruction between scans. Multiplanar reconstruction permits reorientation of CT data in other planes, typically coronal or sagittal.

Three-dimensional (3-D) imaging is a useful technique in evaluating complex fractures of the spine, pelvis, shoulder, and face [4] and in doing reconstructive plastic surgery. Helical (spiral) imaging is used in imaging the chest and abdomen with particular emphasis on liver imaging. Helical imaging allows reduction of contrast and achieves excellent images at the peak of contrast enhancement. Helical scanning also allows the system to obtain improved assessment of vascular anatomy and abnormalities through CT angiography, which is achievable with contrast material. Reconstruction of overlapping sections allows small structures to be seen.

Magnetic Resonance Imaging (MRI)

MRI differs in imaging technique from other modalities in radiology. In x-ray we are imaging the attenuated x-ray passing through the body; in ultrasound, we are imaging the reflected sound wave. In MRI, the body is placed in a magnetic field, and the body part is exposed to a radiofrequency pulse. This causes nuclei in the body to absorb energy. The radio frequency is switched off, and the nuclei continue to emit their excess energy as radiofrequency radiation that can be detected as a signal.

MRI has become a modality very useful in imaging the heart, large blood vessels, brain, and soft tissue masses. MRI can image in transverse, coronal, and sagittal planes and can also show vascular patency without the need for contrast materials.

Recent advances in MRI include the use of contrast material and fast scanning techniques. Magnetic resonance (MR) angiography is a new technique that is gaining recognition, and MR breast imaging is beginning to gain acceptance. Investigations are underway in the area of coupling MR spectroscopy with MR imaging to locate precisely the source of in vivo metabolic activity [4].

When the practice of radiology began with use of the x-ray, it would have been difficult to imagine the various imaging modalities that are common in medical practice today.

▶ ISSUES OF PERCEPTIONS

You may wonder why we are interested in issues of perception. Currently, teaching self-esteem is one of the major thrusts in formal education as well as in the self-help industry. The particular thrust of this book is to present such a strong image of the professional role of the radiographer that, as students leave the classroom and enter the various pathways of the health-care delivery system, they will not develop or be affected by misperceptions of that role. Later, in Chapter 8, we will discuss issues of perceptions in detail. For now, we will look at an image that emerges from Harris's [6] description of the first technicians.

> The dilemma of the doctor—whether in small town middle America or metropolitan New York—remained the same. More and more of his time was eaten up by the mechanics of the x-ray, leaving less time for patient contact and treatment. . . . Physicians such as general practitioners, surgeons, and even radiologists realized that to make the most effective use of their x-ray equipment, someone else had to handle the time-consuming tasks of taking and developing the x-ray films.
>
> The task most often fell to the physician's office assistants. Across the country physicians recruited their secretaries and receptionists to crank the handle of the static machine, pose as subjects and rock the developer pan. . . . The vast majority were women, and they were expected not only to operate the x-ray equipment, but also to perform routine maintenance and repair minor breakdowns. These assistants usually had no knowledge of human anatomy or illness. . . . Physicians lucky enough to employ nurses quickly put them to work as x-ray technicians, for they at least had medical training.
>
> The role of the technicians as an x-ray operator or "manipulator" might best be compared to that of the military conscript—enlisted without warning, and often without choice if they cared to continue

receiving a paycheck—suddenly thrust into a duty that was foreign and, even for the trained nurse, somewhat frightening [6, pp. 19–20].

The most striking feature of Harris's image of the early technician is that it has almost nothing whatsoever to do with the professional role of radiographer as it is currently practiced. The ghosts of these conscripted technicians may, however, still linger in the perceived image of the modern radiographer. Other non-physician health-care professionals have had little difficulty transcending perceptions of their early roles; for example, nurses have no problem being viewed as much more than handmaidens to physicians and physical therapists as much more than masseurs. The primary thrust of other health-care disciplines to gain respect and professional recognition has come largely from advanced education and definition of their professional role.

How we are perceived by others influences how we perceive ourselves. Thus, the issue of perceptions is meaningful to the fledgling radiographer as he or she begins to internalize an image of the radiographer's professional role.

TEST QUESTIONS

1. Radiologists first used "technicians" or assistants for taking test x-rays.
   a. true
   b. false

2. Both radiologists and radiographers share the same professional role; only their educational backgrounds differ.
   a. true
   b. false

3. The professional roles of nurses and radiographers both include elements related to providing patient care services.
   a. true
   b. false

4. Radiographers are, in a sense, artists because of the relationship of producing a radiographic image to:
   a. electricity
   b. magnetism
   c. photography
   d. cave painting
   e. line drawing

5. The profession of radiography relates most closely to the _____ branch of medicine.
   a. preventive
   b. diagnostic
   c. therapeutic
   d. all of the above
   e. none of the above

6. _____ was responsible for developing the first fluoroscope.
   a. Becquerel
   b. Curie
   c. Edison
   d. Compton
   e. Eastman

7. The person primarily responsible for identifying the role of the radiographer (as a technician) in 1922 was:
   a. Coolidge

   b. Jerman
   c. Snook
   d. Lawrence
   e. Rutherford

8. Formal education in radiographic techniques largely evolved from the foundation laid by Wilhem Conrad Röntgen.
   a. true
   b. false

9. The initial organization established to provide national certification for radiographers was recognized in early _____.
   a. 1920
   b. 1922
   c. 1923
   d. 1924
   e. 1925

10. Radiologic technologists have historically experienced strong linkages with representatives of equipment manufacturers and photographic suppliers.
   a. true
   b. false

11. The early title of technician was changed to technologist to reflect new and advanced technologies in the radiologic sciences in the _____.
   a. 1980s
   b. 1970s
   c. 1960s
   d. 1950s
   e. 1940s

12. Match the terms in Column A with the appropriate terms in Column B.

Column A	Column B
1. nuclear medicine	a. echoes
2. mammography	b. radiofrequency pulse
3. ultrasound	c. radionuclides
4. MRI	d. breast imaging

13. Match the scientist(s) in Column A with the discovery/theory in Column B.

Column A
1. Faraday and Henry
2. Volta
3. Hittorf
4. Oersted
5. Ohm

Column B
a. electromagnetic induction
b. cathode rays
c. electricity and magnetism
d. first electric battery
e. formulated laws about the relations between electric current, electromotive force, and resistance.

14. Certification of technicians first began in November _____.
    a. 1950
    b. 1942
    c. 1935
    d. 1927
    e. 1922

15. Match the year in Column A with the term in Column B related to an event which took place in that year.

Column A
1. 1920
2. 1921
3. 1929
4. 1934
5. 1964

Column B
a. *The X-ray Technician*
b. AART
c. first AART meeting
d. ASRT
e. ASXT

▶ REFERENCES

1. Anderson, KN, Anderson, LE. Mosby's pocket dictionary of medicine, nursing, & allied health. St. Louis: Mosby-Year Book, 1994.

2. Bushong, SC. Radiologic science for technologists. 5th ed. St. Louis: Mosby-Year Book, 1993.

3. Bushong, SC. Radiologic science for technologists. 6th ed. St. Louis: Mosby-Year Book, 1997.

4. Eisenberg, RL. Radiology: an illustrated history. St. Louis: Mosby-Year Book, 1997.

5. Glasser, O, Quimby, EH, Taylor, LS, Weatherwax, JL, Morgan, RH. Physical foundations of radiology. 3rd ed. New York: Harper & Row, 1965.

6. Harris, EL. The shadowmakers: a history of radiologic technology. Albuquerque, NM: American Society of Radiologic Technologists, 1995.

7. Seeram, E. Computed tomography: physical principles, clinical application, and quality control. Philadelphia: W. B. Saunders Company, 1994.

8. Stanfield, PS. Introduction to the health professions. 2nd ed. Boston: Jones and Bartlett, 1995.

9. Thomas, EL, ed. Taber's cyclopedic medical dictionary. Philadelphia: F. A. Davis, 1993.

CHAPTER

2

The Hospital Health-Care Team

▶ OBJECTIVES

At the conclusion of the learning opportunity the reader will be able to:

1. Discuss Pellegrino's definition of the patient-centered team and name its subunits.
2. Discuss the components of the Campeau health-care team and explain how they relate to Pellegrino's definition.
3. Explain differences between Pellegrino's concept of the patient-centered team and the patient-centered team as it is often conceptualized today.
4. Identify which health-care professionals are members of the same team as radiographers.
5. Discuss the nature of the relationship between physicians and radiographers.
6. Discuss the characteristics of the relationship between nurses and radiographers.
7. Discuss features of the relationship between radiographers and other technologists.

▶ DEFINITION OF THE HEALTH-CARE TEAM

In the first chapter we examined the professional role of the radiographer (x-ray technician, then radiologic technologist) and traced the emergence and evolution of both radiology and radiologic technology as distinct health professional disciplines. In this chapter we will concentrate on other health-care disciplines but will condense the subject matter so that it encompasses only those professions with which radiographers have frequent contact, especially in the context of participation in the health-care team. It may be prudent to note at this point that although many of the practitioners discussed in this chapter, as well as departments related to their disciplines, can also be found in medical offices and clinics, the intention herein is to discuss the *hospital* health-care team specifically.

Radiographers have been members of the health-care delivery system since the early 1920s when certification of technicians by the Registry organization began. Radiographers thus have a long history of working with other hospital health-care providers. The actual identification of groups of persons involved in the delivery of health care as teams began in the latter half of the twentieth century. For the purposes of this chapter, we will first take a step backward in time to look at the health-care team approach as it was defined in the 1970s and 1980s. During the 1990s the concept of the health-care team has been slanted away from an earlier patient-care orientation and toward a cost-containment outcome. This latter outcome involves cross-training health-care professionals from one discipline in skills practiced by other disciplines. This change of focus may or may not prove lasting—although it might be cost effective, quality-of-care issues remain in question.

In 1972 Pellegrino wrote, "The purpose of a team approach is to optimize the special contribution in skills and knowledge of the team members so that the needs of the persons served can be met more efficiently, competently, and more considerately than would be possible by independent and individual action" [1, p. 6]. Pellegrino also defined "two types of teams, functional and patient centered. Both are transitory and both depend on the problem to be solved. . . . Functional teams are those whose personnel depend on the nature of the problem. . . . Patient-centered teams are made up in terms of closeness of patient contact" [1, p. 6]. Pellegrino identified three types of patient-centered teams: the patient care team, the medical care team, and the health care team (see Figure 2-1). Under his definition, the professional role of radiologic technologists places them in the medical care team—people "who provide 'essential back-up services for the patient care teams . . . not in close continual contact with the patient . . . some deal transiently on a personal basis with the patient . . . for a short interval'" [1, pp. 6–7]. In Pellegrino's view, the patient-care team includes people "'who jointly provide needed services that bring them into direct personal and physical contact with the patient and which are part of his personal and individualized program of management.' These are . . . doctors, nurses, therapists and so forth" [1, p. 6]. The health-care team in this design "is made up of persons who are the 'most distantly related to the individual patients and usually have as their concern the entire community . . . (this group includes) public health officers, hospital administrators, health educators, bio-medical engineers, sanitarians, etc.'" [1, p. 7].

Terminology has changed considerably since Pellegrino described the teams commonly found in hospitals in 1972. However, his overarching concept of the purpose of patient-oriented health-

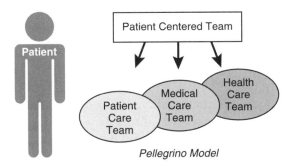

Pellegrino Model

FIGURE 2-1. Pellegrino's model of the patient-centered team includes three categories: patient-care team (closest contact with patient), medical-care team (provision of essential back-up services and/or intermittent contact with patient), health-care team (public health personnel, regulators, health administrators, etc.). (*Source:* Adapted by Carol Cornette.)

care teams is as valid today as it was then. Although this chapter will use Pellegrino's description of the patient-centered team as the basis for the discussion of specific health professions, the term *health-care team*, rather than patient-centered team, will be used as the name for the collective patient-centered group. This model, herein called the Campeau model, is illustrated in Figure 2-2. The term health-care team is commonly used and understood today as the team Pellegrino defined as patient-centered team. In recent years, the meaning of the

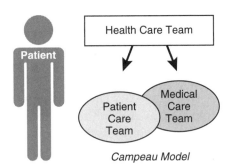

Campeau Model

FIGURE 2-2. Campeau's model of the health-care team includes two of Pellegrino's categories, the patient-care team and the medical-care team. This model, viewed as one unit, reflects the most commonly accepted design for the interdisciplinary health-care team during the 1970s, 1980s, and early 1990s. (*Source:* Adapted by Carol Cornette.)

term *patient-centered care* has been narrowed to a particular kind of health-care delivery, which will be discussed in the context of Chapters 3 (the health care delivery system) and 4 (the hospital radiology department). Pellegrino's differentiation between the patient-care team and the medical-care team remains valid today. Thus, definitions of terms used in this chapter are as follows:

> *Health-care team*: Members are determined in "terms of closeness of patient contact" [1]. This collective team is divided into two separate subsets.
>
> *Patient-care team*: Members (physicians, nurses, therapists) lay hands directly on patients, have the most sustained contact with them as people, and provide individualized services related to the program of care [1].
>
> *Medical-care team*: Members provide "essential back-up services (e.g., diagnostic tests, pharmaceuticals) for the patient-care teams" but have only transient contact with patients for short periods of time (e.g., radiographers) or perform tests without necessarily making personal contact (medical technologists) [1].

▶ RADIOGRAPHERS AS MEMBERS OF THE HEALTH-CARE TEAM

When people become ill and lose control over their health, they also lose their autonomy and must depend on others to help restore them, if possible, to a state of well-being and independence. Members of the health-care team (doctors, nurses, and various technologists and assistants) all contribute to the patient's diagnosis, treatment, and, possibly, reattainment of health.

During the past thirty years, patient and quality-of-care issues have been balanced against cost-of-care issues; in view of escalating health care costs, it has been impossible not to give some weight to the cost-of-care side. Health care institutions, agencies, and providers have all had to rethink how they can do business in terms of efficiency and cost effectiveness and yet deliver quality care. The team approach to health-care delivery has gained steadily in importance as the system has undergone change. The team approach itself has undergone change in efforts to provide quality care to patients but in a way that is cost effective for the hospital or agency.

A radiologic technologist is an image maker—the end product of the various modalities is provision of information through imaging that otherwise is not available without more invasive procedures. The radiographer's relationship with other members of the health-care team is critical to the work performed by the medical team as well as to quality care for the patient. The various people with whom radiographers routinely work in hospitals and offices are physicians, nurses, other imaging technologists, and technologists from other disciplines. All of these people must be respected for the job they do and the professional roles they have been educated and trained to fill—each job and role requires specific knowledge and skills and carries with it specific areas of initiative/authority and responsibility. In the first chapter brief definitions of the various imaging modalities were presented. Discussion in this chapter will focus on physicians, nurses, and other technologists with whom radiographers are frequently in contact and on the relationship of radiographers to these other disciplines. The main point of emphasis in considering the relationships among health-care practitioners is that it is important for each discipline to recognize and have respect for the professional roles, particular areas of expertise, and scopes of practice of the other disciplines and to work compatibly with others within the boundaries of the scope of practice of the individual member's discipline.

Physicians' Relationship to Radiographers

A physician is "a health professional who has earned a degree of Doctor of Medicine (MD) after completing an approved course of study at an approved medical school," satisfactorily completing National Board Examinations, and completing one year of post-graduate training (internship) or completing further training in a specialty [2, p. 816]. Physicians are required to be licensed in the state where they practice. It is the physician who has ultimate responsibility for patient care, treatment, and outcome. The choice of treatment is generally contingent upon one or many diagnostic tests performed to assist the physician in completing a diagnosis based on concurrent findings from physical and visual examination of the patient. Many professional practitioners—physicians, nurses, technologists, clergy, social workers—as well as clerical workers and varying levels of medical assistants may come in contact with patients in order to meet their holistic medical needs in a course of treatment. It is the physician, however, who is team leader because he or she is the one who makes the primary commitment in the patient/physician contract.

The professional relationship between the physician and the radiographer is determined largely through the fact that the radiographer follows the physician's orders, that is, the radiographer performs the procedures a physician has ordered. These procedures must be performed according to the physician's direction, yet within the boundaries set by the code of ethics outlined by the American Society of Radiology Technologists. This code will be addressed in some detail in Chapters 8 and 9; however, the first and sixth items are particularly relevant to the present discussion.

1. The Radiologic Technologist conducts himself/herself in a professional manner, responds to patient needs and supports colleagues and associates in providing quality patient care.
6. The Radiologic Technologist acts as an agent through observation and communication to obtain pertinent information for the physician to aid in the diagnosis and treatment management of the patient, and recognizes that interpretation and diagnosis are outside the scope of practice for the profession. (ASRT)

Additionally, one element of the radiographer's professional role—technically competent practitioner—especially relates to the relationship of the physician and the radiographer. The physician depends on the radiographer to provide the visual information (image) needed in the diagnostic evaluation of a patient; the information in the radiographic image must be anatomically correct and free of artifacts and motion so there is no doubt about its accuracy when it is read. On the other hand, radiographers can expect that they not be given orders to perform in such a way that their professional ethics are challenged or breached. The relationship between the physician and the radiographer involves written and oral communications as well as elements of human respect and professional courtesy.

Nurses' Relationship to Radiographers

A simple definition of a nurse is "an individual who provides health care. The extent of participation varies from simple patient-care tasks to the most expert professional techniques necessary in acute life-threatening situations" [3, p. 1328]. The scope of practice just described implies a range of preparation for a nursing career starting at the level of practical nurse training and terminating at an earned university doctoral degree. The professional role of nurses is described in some detail in nursing literature; some elements of that role relating to patient care and advocacy are similar to the radiographer's professional role. Remember that nurses, along with physicians, belong to the patient-care team and that radiographers are members of the medical-care team. The difference between the two teams rests in the degree to which members of the two teams are in direct personal and physical contact with patients and provide services that are part of patients' personal and individualized programs of management.

Radiographers in hospitals come in general contact with associate degree and baccalaureate degree nurses (registered nurses) as well as practical nurses or nurses' aides. Master's level nurses usually work in supervisory or management roles or in specialty areas; radiographers have less contact with this level of nurse and rarely have contact with doctorally prepared nurses. It is important for radiographers to coordinate their work with the work of nurses wherever coordination is pertinent. If, for example, the physician orders radiographs, the nurse must make sure that the radiology department is contacted and that the patient is sent to the department or the procedure is done by a portable x-ray unit. Coordination is important because nurses are responsible for the first line of care for the hospitalized patient; that is, the nurse, as a member of the patient-care team responsible for the patient's personal and individualized program of management, must assure that the patient's needs are met. Nurses make observations and perform assessments of the patient's physical, mental, emotional, social, and spiritual condition and develop care plans for the level of care nursing provides. They manage the day-to-day care of the hospitalized patient, but the physician is the leader of the team who directs the patient's care.

In some situations, as in surgery and emergency units, radiographers may participate to a greater extent in the patient-care team activities than they do in the radiology department. The relationship between the nurse and the radiographer, similar to that of the physician and radiographer, involves written and oral communications as well as elements of human respect and professional courtesy.

Other Technologists' Relationship to Radiographers

Radiographers are not the only technologists who perform diagnostic or therapeutic procedures for patients. Personnel in the general category of technologists include other imaging technologists—radiographers usually share space in the radiology department with these technologists. Other members of the diagnostic medical-care team include medical technologists, pathologists, and pharmacists. Within the hospital environment and as fellow members of the medical-care team, radiographers do have contact with medical technologists. Radiographers ordinarily do not have professional contact with pathologists nor with pharmacists. Thus, the remainder of this section will deal with other imaging technologists and medical technologists.

Radiology Department

Nuclear Medicine Technologists.   Education in nuclear medicine technology is grounded in the physical sciences, as is education for radiologic technology. Both disciplines use diagnostic imaging equipment for performing their work. In radiography the image is produced by making exposures (images that look like negatives) of a particular part of the human anatomy. In nuclear medicine technology, however, radioactive substances, or pharmaceuticals, are administered to the patient either orally or by injection. Nuclear medicine procedures must be completed within a given time period because the radioactive substances have a half-life (the substance loses its radioactivity within a specified time period—30 minutes, one hour, 3 hours, etc.). This half-life factor is what makes the use of radioactive substances possible for human diagnostic purposes.

Radiographers and nuclear medicine technologists often share a basic educational background in the physical sciences. These two disciplines have been linked educationally since the 1960s. Initially, most nuclear medicine technologists were first radiographers, and it became accepted practice for nuclear medicine technology to be considered advanced education for radiographers. Although this approach is still available today, education and technology have created totally separate curriculum systems so that many nuclear medicine technologists have no professional background in radiography and vice versa. However, the professional roles of the two technology disciplines are essentially the same—in fact, if technologists are credentialed in both radiography and nuclear medicine technology, they may be assigned to work in both areas. The relationship of radiographers and nuclear medicine technologists in the hospital environment is basically one of colleagues or peers.

Diagnostic Medical Sonographers. Practitioners of this imaging modality are also called ultrasonographers; ultrasound may be a more commonly recognized name for the modality. Indeed, *ultrasound* has become something of a household word since a large number of pregnant women in the United States receive an ultrasound study of the fetus in utero to determine if any growth or development problems exist; in many cases the parents wish to know the sex of the developing fetus.

Very specialized equipment is used to produce images through the sonography method. Specific uses were mentioned in the first chapter. Ultrasound began gaining in popularity in the 1970s and was added to most radiology departments in hospitals, although some sonography units have been established separate from imaging departments in hospitals and mobile units. The educational background of ultrasonographers is very broad. As in radiography and nuclear medicine technology, the sonographer must have a background in the physical sciences. Often, sonographers are nurses, radiographers, nuclear medicine technologists, or various other allied health professionals who have received education and training in sonography either through formal education programs or through on-the-job training and have gained credentials in sonography. Again, the professional roles of the radiographer and the sonographer follow, for the most part, parallel lines. However, the sonographer's role does not include elements related to radiation safety and protection; no significant undesirable biological effects related to sonography have been identified.

Thus, the relationship of radiographers and sonographers in the hospital environment is basically one of colleagues or peers.

Other Imaging Modalities. Three other imaging modalities—mammography, magnetic resonance imaging (MRI), and computed tomography (CT)—are either housed in the hospital radiology department or the equipment is housed in a separate department but is generally operated by radiographers with advanced training. Mammography space is generally allocated in the hospital radiology department. The equipment must be operated by radiographers who are certified in mammography and who must meet federal regulations for mammography. CT equipment is frequently located outside the radiology department; MRI equipment always is. Equipment for these two modalities, similar to equipment used in radiation therapy, requires amounts of space and, often, special housing that precludes its placement in a radiology department. Radiographers can receive certification as operators of CT and MRI equipment also. General radiographers' relationships with radiographers who operate mammography, CT, and MRI equipment is that of colleagues and peers.

Medical Technologists' Relationship with Radiographers

Medical technologists in the hospital work in clinical pathology laboratories. Medical technologists hold or are eligible to hold a baccalaureate degree and must become registered to practice. They work in a variety of specialized areas, including microbiology, parasitology, blood and body fluid chemistry, toxicology, immunology, immunohematology, urinalysis, and hematology. Collection of samples for analysis in the hospital is most frequently done by practitioners other than the medical technologists themselves. Their paths rarely cross with radiographers in day-to-day activities. Occasionally, a medical technologist may need to draw blood while a patient is in radiology. More likely, the radiographer may have to wait for the medical techologist to complete his or her work before the imaging procedure is begun (e.g, when films are taken at bedside by portable equipment).

▶ CHANGES IN THE HEALTH-CARE TEAM

Along with the development of a type of health-care delivery called patient-centered care in which nurse and technologist level practitioners are cross-trained in other disciplines, some radiographers have been called upon to step outside the boundaries of their traditional role and expand their educational base and skills. It is unclear at this time whether the patient-centered care concept is one that will be validated as reasonable and useful when it is applied in practice over time. However, radiographers need to acknowledge the fact that they may be required to adapt to new methodologies of delivering close and personal patient care if they want to remain full participants in the hospital health-care delivery system. If they become members of the patient-centered care team as it is practiced today, their professional role and scope of practice will undergo change and they may have contact with additional health-care providers not addressed in this chapter.

TEST QUESTIONS

1. The most commonly accepted design for the health-care team during the 1970s, 1980s, and early 1990s consisted of a patient-care team and a medical-care team.
   a. true
   b. false

2. Relationships among health-care practitioners is important. Practitioners of each discipline must recognize and respect their own and other disciplines':
   a. scopes of practice
   b. areas of expertise
   c. professional roles
   d. a and b
   e. a, b, and c

3. Given the ASRT Code of Ethics for Radiographers, which of the following principles (codes) are most relevant to the professional relationship between radiographers and physicians?
   a. 1
   b. 2
   c. 6
   d. a and c
   e. b and c

4. The principles identified in question 3 address guidelines involving the radiographer's role in:
   1. achieving technical competence
   2. responding to patient needs
   3. supporting colleagues and associates in providing quality patient care
   4. obtaining pertinent patient information for the physician to aid in diagnosis and treatment management
      a. 1 and 4
      b. 2 and 3
      c. 1, 2 and 3
      d. 2, 3, and 4
      e. all of the above

35

5. One of the differences between physicians and nurses and radiographers rests in the degree that each is in direct personal and physical contact with the patient and is responsible for management of the patient's care.
   a. true
   b. false

6. Areas in which the radiographer's role may be expanded to first-line contact with the patient are:
   a. surgery
   b. emergency units
   c. patient management
   d. a and b
   e. all of the above

7. Radiographers generally have little or no contact with hospital health-care members who are:
   a. other imaging technologists
   b. pharmacists
   c. pathologists
   d. a and b
   e. b and c

8. Match the terms in Column A with the most relevant practitioner in Column B.

   Column A
   a. pregnant women
   b. observes and assesses
      patient needs
   c. radioactive substances
   d. interacts directly with
      other imaging technologists
   e. patient management

   Column B
   1. radiographer
   2. nuclear medicine technologist
   3. nurse
   4. ultrasonographer
   5. physician

9. Which of the following disciplines share a similar educational background in the physical sciences?
   a. radiography
   b. ultrasonography
   c. nuclear medicine technology
   d. a and c
   e. a, b, and c

10. Diagnostic medical sonographers are required to have _____ hours of education in radiation safety and biological effects.
    a. 15 hours
    b. 30 hours
    c. 10 hours
    d. 0 hours
    e. none of the above

11. Diagnostic medical sonographers are generally credentialed health-care professionals from:
    a. nursing
    b. radiography
    c. other allied health disciplines
    d. a and b
    e. a, b, and c

12. Procedures performed by _____, as opposed to other specialty areas in radiology, are the only radiological procedures where federal regulations require the radiographers to be certified.
    a. sonography
    b. mammography
    c. nuclear medicine technology
    d. magnetic resonance imaging
    e. computed tomography

13. The health-care discipline that performs very important analyses in a variety of specialized areas, but has a limited amount of direct contact with the patient is:
    a. nuclear medical technology
    b. medical technology
    c. radiography
    d. medicine
    e. nursing

14. Radiographers are identified within the health-care team as members of the:
    a. patient-care team
    b. medical-care team

15. According to the Pellegrino model, the health-care team is determined in relationship to closeness of patient contact.
    a. true
    b. false

▶ REFERENCES

1. Allen, AS (Ed.). (1980). *Introduction to health professions* (3rd ed.). St. Louis: The C. V. Mosby Company.

2. Anderson, KN, Anderson, LE. (Eds.) (1994). *Mosby's pocket dictionary of medicine, nursing, and allied health* (2nd ed.). St Louis: The C. V. Mosby Company.

3. Thomas, EL (Ed.). (1993). *Taber's cyclopedic medical dictionary*. Philadelphia: F. A. Davis Company.

CHAPTER

Health-Care Delivery System/Hospitals

▶ OBJECTIVES

At the conclusion of the learning opportunity the reader will be able to:

1. Discuss the structure of health-care delivery.
2. Provide an overview of medical care from the early 1900s to health-care reform in the late 1900s.
3. Define three levels of health-care delivery.
4. Discuss the general philosophy of the hospital as an institution.

▶ STRUCTURE

In the United States, *health-care delivery system* is an expression used to encompass the many parts of the structure that provides traditional health care—preventive, diagnostic, and therapeutic—to the public. Everyone and every occupation involved in providing such care plays a role in the overall organization of the system. Thus, hospital administrators, physicians, dentists, nurses, physical therapists, medical technologists, cytotechnologists, physical therapist assistants, practical nurses, medical assistants, and so forth, are all small subsystems operating within the larger one. To name all the professions and occupations functioning as part of the health-care delivery system would be a daunting task for author and reader. Let us note here, however, that radiography is a profession very important in the overall system.

Institutionalization of health care as a system commenced in the United States in the mid-nineteenth century with the appearance of large hospitals such as Bellevue in New York, Cook County in Chicago, and Massachusetts General in Boston. Initially, only scattered independent and unrelated services were available. In its present state the traditional health-care delivery system is conceived as offering care at three levels—primary care, secondary care, and tertiary care. Briefly, the system is thus divided according to where the client is provided care—a physician's office or primary care center, a local hospital, or a large regional hospital. However, the development of managed care during the past twenty-five years has greatly changed the pattern of health-care delivery. Because many health maintenance organizations have primary care centers that offer a broader scope of services than are ordinarily available in a physician's office, the boundaries separating the primary and secondary levels of care may be blurring to some extent. The traditional three levels of care, as well as managed care, will be discussed in more detail later in the chapter.

Alternative forms of health care have received increasing acceptance by the public within the past decade. Such modalities as healing touch, massage therapy, acupuncture, aroma therapy, herbal and homeopathic supplements, vitamin and mineral supplements, meditation, tai chi, yoga, to name a few, have become increasingly recognized by some segments of the population as viable options to consider in the pursuit of attaining and/or maintaining well-being. Such forms of health care have gained in popularity and acceptance and some forms have proven to be legitimate and effective. Accordingly, the traditional view of the health-care delivery system may have to be altered somewhat to accomodate them; in some future time, it may be necessary to expand the concept of the health-care delivery system to include a fourth level, that of self-health care and other alternative forms of medicine.

For the purposes of this chapter, the health-care delivery system will be viewed as integrally aligned to services provided by physicians because the present system, although it includes the services of the other helping professions, evolved largely through the practice of medicine. The system we are discussing involves hospitals at the secondary and tertiary care levels. First, we will briefly examine the system from three perspectives: development of health care in the United States from the mid-1800s to the present, medical practice reform, and financing health care; next, we will take a look at the three levels of care in the present day delivery system, including managed care; and, finally, we will examine the philosophy, mission and goals, and organization of the standard U.S. hospital.

Development

Mid-19th Century to Early 1900s.   In whatever fashion the public benefitted from any type of very early medical care in the United States, the aims of the medical community at large were primarily to satisfy the economic woes of society by getting people well and back to work or to make the distasteful conditions of disease more obscure by placing victims collectively—aged, orphaned, mentally ill, physically ill—in almshouses or poor houses. These institutions generally served welfare needs while providing incidental care for illness [13].

The early practice of medicine in America attempted to change the course of disease by "sweating, blistering, purging, and bleeding" the body [14]. Many of these techniques carried over until the late 1800s and early 1900s when medical research began to emerge through educational revisions.

Until the mid-1800s, when physicians began to seek control of medical education in the United States, collective professional concerns dealt mostly with medical practitioners' fees rather than with their skills [14]. However, physicians were not so much driven by profit as by obligation to come to the aid of society's frailties [2].

There were many medical schools after 1812 [13] with a myriad of conflicting and competing interests. However, a common theme across the nation among eastern schools, western schools, local medical societies, and the public in general was hostility toward fee schedules.

One of the most important and significant changes in health care came with the formation in 1847 of a medical society, which would later become the American Medical Association (AMA). (This society/association will be referred to as *AMA* henceforth in this chapter.) The early goals of the AMA were to establish an organization of regular doctors (allopaths). Their concern was primarily that of acquiring control of medicine from laymen by developing a single, unified society of educated physicians. The AMA was not to become effective as a national organization until the demise of medical college voting authority and recognition of the AMA at the local, county, and state levels in 1902.

The Civil War period brought some shortcomings of medical practice into sharp focus. Doctors could combat infection only by amputation of body parts and by fierce debridement of wounds. The magnitude of pain accompanying such procedures led to extensive testing of the anesthetics ether and chloroform in the battlefields and nearby surgeries.

Following the Civil War, the practice of medicine began a growth period that included specialization and significant changes in medical education and public awareness. Many hospitals began to emerge in larger cities.

Some of the earliest specialties were established between the 1820s and the 1860s; eye and ear, lying-in hospitals, and skin disease all had become specialties. Care of the mentally ill was a major medical concern at this time. The public was becoming aware of the need to separate the mentally ill from the often wretched conditions housing victims of infectious and chronic diseases.

The evolution of medical specialties strengthened and gave credence to improvements in medical education and helped to create legislative regulation of medical practice. Initial concerns did not deal so much with patient/physician relationships as with concerns of professional integrity among physicians; efforts at this time on the part of the AMA to establish standards of practice dealt with the general behavior of physicians toward each other.

Formation of the AMA, as well as its increase in prominence and influence through the mid-1800s to the early 1900s, led to establishment of the organization that has had the greatest impact on medical practice. It also created division among politicians, laymen, and philanthropists.

The next major period in medicine began in the early 1900s when medical education received a severe attack in the Abraham Flexner report of 1910. Issues regarding methods of treatment and patient/physician relationship would soon evolve.

Medical Practice Reform.   Until about 1900 the practice of medicine largely dealt with infectious conditions, often of epidemic proportions. There was almost no technology available to educate physicians; only theorized techniques for avoiding disease were promoted, for example, fresh air or techniques for purging the body of disease. Generally, health care was provided in the home and patients were visited by their physicians. However, if hospitalization became necessary, they were isolated from other patients and provided preferential treatment.

After the Civil War, U.S. cities were growing, technology was increasing communications through the telegraph and railroads [14], and medicine was beginning to reform. Although there had been a proliferation of schools offering medical education, instruction was not like the education received in medical school today. Often it was more of an apprenticeship than an academic program.

Two institutions had a profound impact on medical education: Johns Hopkins Medical School, which opened in 1893, and the

Carnegie Foundation, through the Flexner report. The Johns Hopkins school developed medical education as a graduate program that included patient and laboratory facilities, upgraded admission standards, and clinical instruction based on the German model from full-time professors. Johns Hopkins medical students had to have an AB degree or equivalent with language and certain premedical studies, and the school established a 4-year clinical curriculum with preprofessional requirements. Developments of Johns Hopkins Hospital (1889) and a nursing school further distinguished the program as a scientific model for education of physicians.

The second major event in educational reform occurred when Abraham Flexner, a Johns Hopkins University graduate and established professional educator, was commissioned by the Carnegie Foundation to investigate professional education in medical schools throughout the United States and Canada.

Flexner visited all 155 medical programs in the United States and Canada. His inspection included laboratory and equipment resources, faculty qualifications, student capacity, admissions criteria, curriculum, clinical facilities with patient teaching material, and endowment support [3]. Because the study was initiated by the AMA Council on Medical Education and financed by the Carnegie Foundation, all schools were forced to cooperate with Flexner's investigation; otherwise they risked loss of credibility and support from the AMA. Prior to the Flexner report (1910), the AMA was promoting centralized control of medical education and the practice of medicine.

Too many doctors were being produced, especially from commercial schools. Overcrowding provided motivation to control practice through increasingly medical education standards. The notion was that fewer, better qualified doctors were needed.

Flexner's report agreed with an earlier assessment of AMA officials that schools were overcrowded and did not have adequate facilities and faculty. Also, it was Flexner's perception that medicine was so intertwined with the social structure that doctors were obligated to maintain a professional image that set them apart from and above anyone else.

As a recognized educator, Flexner focused the major thrust of his report on standardizing the medical curriculum so that it would have educational consistency. This, he concluded, would improve the social status of the medical profession.

Along with social changes, the technology awareness emerging from the Civil War, and standardization of medical education, ethical standards also were undergoing revision by the AMA. The first Code of Ethics, adopted in 1847, included few patient concerns (the patient was only expected to obey) in favor of more intra-professional concerns. The first revision of the code in 1903 offered an extensive set of "Principles of Medical Ethics" from which each state or associated society could develop its own guidelines for standards of professional conduct based on religion and morals [8]. Specific problems, such as fee splitting between surgeons and referring physicians, were not yet addressed.

It was not until 1955 that revision of the code began to include such terms as fees, consultation, and confidentiality. Prior to these changes, the AMA principles were written more in a suggestive or advisory nature, using terms like *should* or *ought to*. The 1980 code began to mandate certain behavior of physicians; the term *shall* precedes all written statements.

In summary, while social and educational reforms were underway, physicians (the AMA) required appropriate behavioral adjustments. The Hippocratic paternalistic philosophy was not compatible with the holistic changes evolving in society. As technical care improved, patients' rights and truth telling were to become the modern buzz words.

Financing Health Care: Then and Now.   From the Revolutionary War through the period following the Civil War, the practice of medicine was conducted in many forms. However, no matter what approach was taken to help the sick—regular, homeopathic, eclectic, quackery—all were limited in knowledge and success. Rather than relying on methods quickly becoming dated, medicine needed to become firmly grounded in the scientific realm, which was expanding by leaps and bounds. Without the recognition by the Flexner report of 1910 of the relationship of basic sciences to medical education and the subsequent need for hospital standards to assure quality education, modern medical technology might have taken much longer to develop.

Since the Civil War and the gradual increase in medical technology and education, particularly in surgical and specialty areas, the cost of medical care has concurrently increased. Resources for expansion and construction, sophisticated medical technology and computed hospital care, power of unions, and the hospitals' limited power to control physician practice are some of the reasons the hospital industry has continued to have cost containment problems [16].

The concept of health insurance began around 1915 as a movement based on the ideal of social guarantees for an efficient and healthy worker population. By 1920, largely because of confusion over its value, the health insurance movement had lost its energy and was dead. By 1940 group hospitalization prepayment plans (e.g., Blue Cross) had become typical for many hospitals over the nation [15]. This effort was energized after World War II through government intervention. Institutionalization of the entitlement programs medicare and Medicaid by 1966 stands as a landmark in the history of government health insurance. In the 1970s national health insurance became a political imperative [14].

The AMA spent an unprecedented amount of money—nearly one million dollars—lobbying against Medicare in 1965 and lost [11]. At that point health care had become considered more a right and less a fee-for-service privilege.

According to Brown [3], a 1974 Congressional report estimated that there had been 2.4 million unnecessary operations in the United States and that over 11,000 deaths could have been avoided along with a $3.9 billion cost. Through the 1970s surgeons had largely been guilty of filling hospital beds with unnecessary operations for huge fees. It is thus understandable that there was special interest among surgeons and the AMA to fight any type of government intervention into the area of medical costs.

Following the implementation of Medicare during the Johnson administration, the concept of health maintenance was brought to the forefront during the Nixon administration in 1970 [15]. Prepaid group practice was becoming a necessity for physicians, who no longer could claim to be the sole voice of medicine: The public had begun to declare an inalienable right to health care.

The concept of prepaid health maintenance caused all hospitals—voluntary, public, private, and religious—to take a whole new look at hospital management and administrative structure. Between 1965 and 1975 hospital corporations evolved into the multiple institutions that exist today [15].

Health-care planning did not achieve full stride before the 1980s, when the health maintenance organization (HMO) and preferred provider organization (PPO), to mention only two, along with government legislation, were set in place. These programs were designed to limit cost by way of specific choice of physicians and benefits, for example, group practice and diagnostic related group studies (DRGs). Cost limitation in such programs is achieved through control of access to providers, control of benefits available through plans, and control of reimbursement through assignment of patients into case types according to diagnostic categories (DRGs).

It would not seem appropriate to overlook ideas currently emerging regarding the health-care system. As pointed out by McGregor [10], the real culprits in medical costs are technology and allocation of resources. In the past forty years it is not the hospital's external structure that has changed, but the revolution in medicine occurring inside. Doctors no longer carry most of the tools of their trade in a little black bag. McGregor poses an important question: "Is new technology (financially) feasible? . . . Is it worth the cost?" [10]. He charges the medical profession with the responsibility of determining value and cost of new technology based on human welfare and scientific validity and charges the public with the responsibility of making choices based on information.

Financing health care has become an enormous and somewhat disturbing challenge. The question is, Can quality medical care remain a basic right, as opposed to privilege or individual responsibility, as was the case in the early years of Medicare? Related questions are, Where will the money come from? Who will benefit most? How will medical care in its totality continue to be financed?

The decade of the 1990s has been very much occupied by health-care reform thus far. The federal government and many states have taken up the challenge to change the health-care system, but no satisfactory solutions have yet been found to control costs and still provide an acceptable standard level of care to all citizens.

Many public health problems, such as trauma, epidemics of acute infections, chronic systemic diseases (heart disease, cancer, and stroke), and chronic mental diseases and conditions, have existed for many years and continue to exist. However, there are two problems that pose an immediate crisis for health care [7]: access to health-care and acquired immune deficiency syndrome (AIDS).

Nearly 20 percent of the population either lacks a physician, clinic, hospital, or other source of medical care or has great difficulty getting medical care when it is needed [7]. AIDS poses a threat to not only the United States but also many other countries. Although progress has been made in the treatment of AIDS, it may still become widespread because of unchecked cases and because the disease is slow to manifest from the time of infection to the onset of AIDS [7].

Three Levels of Care

Earlier in this chapter we learned that health care is said to be delivered on three levels: primary, secondary, and tertiary. Primary care refers to "the first contact in any given episode of illness that leads to a decision regarding a course of action to resolve the health problem [1]." Secondary health care is "an intermediate level of health care that includes diagnosis and treatment, preferred in a hospital having specialized equipment and laboratory facilities" [1]. Tertiary health care is "a specialized, highly technical level of health care that includes diagnosis and treatment of disease and disability in sophisticated, large research and teaching hospitals. It offers a highly centralized care to the population of a large region, in some cases to the world" [1].

Health-care reform, which began in the early 1970s with businesses and appears to have been more focused at the tertiary health-care level, transformed today's managed care system. Managed care is defined as a system that includes the management of health-care delivery and payment for its services [6]. Managed care and health maintenance organization principles are based on disease prevention and early detection of disease, as opposed to the compensatory fee-for-service approach that paid for every small nuance that physicians and institutions could justify. The economics of managed care/health maintenance organization principles is based on capitation contracts; that is, as providers of health-care services, hospitals and physicians "receive a certain payment per person per month rather than being compensated for each procedure" [6]. In other words, a plan is devised to maximize the cost of health-care delivery to include each member enrolled in the plan, regardless of how much care each member requires. The total amount of care may be determined by identifying a continuum of care for a wide range of services and the extent to which these services will be applied or utilized. Services in-

BOX 3-1   The ABCs of Managed Care

Alliances: One or more regional health provider system(s) established in each state to offer at least basic health-care coverage for all residents in that geographic region.[a]

Alternative Delivery System (ADS): A method of providing health-care benefits that departs from traditional indemnity methods.[a]

Benefit Package: A collection of specific services or benefits that the HMO is obligated to provide under terms of its contracts with subscriber groups or individuals.[a]

Capitation: A per-member, per-month fixed payment to a health-care provider or health plan for each member enrolled, regardless of the amount of care a member requires. The specific services that are covered must be stated.[a]

Capitation, Mixed: This is an agreement that excludes specified services from the agreement. These excluded services are paid for on a fee-for-service basis, with discounts, if any, having been previously negotiated.[a]

Copayment: A set fee paid by the patient for an office visit or other covered service (generally $5 to $15).[b]

Deductible: In traditional health insurance, the amount a patient must pay out of his or her own pocket before coverage kicks in.[b]

Diagnostic Related Groups (DRG): Classification system . . . using 383 major diagnostic categories. . . . This procedure assigns patients into case types.[a]

Fee-for-Service: The traditional form of payment, in which the patient or insurer pays for each doctor visit or service provided.[b]

Group Contract: An agreement between the HMO and a subscribing group specifying rates, performance covenants, relationships among parties, schedule of benefits, and other conditions.[a]

Group Model HMO: Care is provided by a network of physician group practices that have agreed to accept a certain level of payment.[b]

Health Care Financing Administration (HCFA): Part of the U.S. Department of Health and Human Services. . . . HCFA is the contracting agency for HMOs who seek direct contractor/provider status for provisions of the Medicare benefit package.[a]

Health Maintenance Organization (HMO): An organization that finances, organizes, and provides health care using the principles of managed care.[b]

Health Network: HMOs, PPOs, or any cooperative system of insurers, doctors, or hospitals that contracts with employers to provide medical care.[a]

Health Practice Association (HPA) model HMO: A type of HMO in which doctors in private practice are paid to care for health plan members.[b]

BOX 3-1   *Continued*

Managed Care: Use of planned and coordinated approach to providing health care with the goal of quality care at lower cost. Usually emphasizes preventive care and often associated with an HMO.[a]

Mixed Model HMO: A plan that includes more than one model; for example, a staff model HMO might also contract with some group practices or individual physicians to provide care in certain geographic areas. [b]

Per Member Per Month (PMPM): Refers to the cost or revenue from each plan's member for one month. In capitated contracts the provider is reimbursed each month based on the number of enrollees in the plan regardless of the volume of care provided.[a]

Point of Service (POS) plan: Coverage that allows members to use out-of-network services, as long as they pay a deductible and part of the cost.[b]

Preferred Provider Organization (PPO): A network of physicians and hospitals that contract with an insurance company to care for its policyholders at discounted fees.[b]

Primary Care Physician: Provides treatment of routine injuries and illnesses and focuses on preventive care. Services as "gatekeeper" for managed care.[a]

Prior Authorization: Procedure used in managed care to control utilization of services by prospective reviewing and approval requirements before a member can have a service provided.[a]

Service Area: The territory within certain boundaries than an HMO designates for providing service to members.[a]

Staff Model HMO: All care is delivered at HMO-run facilities by salaried staff doctors; also called a "closed panel" plan.[b]

Utilization: The frequency with which a benefit is used, for example, 3200 doctor's office visits per 1000 HMO members per year. Utilization experience multiplied by the average cost per unit service delivered equals the amount that will be a basis to calculate a PMPM rate.[a]

Utilization Review: A program that examines the medical necessity of non-emergency hospital admissions and medical procedures or tests.[a]

---

[a]Definition from "Glossary, Managed Care Terms," 1997, *Radiology Management* 19(2), pp. 7–8, 10–12. Copyright 1996 by Bracco Diagnostics Inc., Princeton, New Jersey. Adapted with permission of the author.

[b]Definition from "Managed Care: Choosing an HMO," by DW Gregg, 1996, *Harvard Health Letter, April (Special Suppl),* p. 10. Copyright 1996 by Harvard Health Letter. Adapted with permission of the author.

clude health care provided to varying age groups, from the very young (who ordinarily need little care) to the elderly (who often need extensive care). Services also include health care provided for varying types of disease/conditions, from simple, short-term to complex, chronic. It is possible for very efficient health-care organizations to keep abreast of reimbursement profit. There is some concern that motivation for profit may result in decision making that has the potential to reduce the quality of care and consequently result in grievous health consequences for the individual member. Many terms are associated with managed care systems; Box 3-1 lists definitions of the most commonly used terms.

The impact of managed care on radiographers will most likely be felt through hospitals and other providers downsizing to reduce costs. This means that in the future radiographers will need to be multicompetent in radiology skills (radiography, computed tomography [CT], magnetic resonance imaging [MRI], and ultrasound) as well as to have enhanced capability in the skill areas of patient care, patient satisfaction, and patient education. The radiologic sciences technologist will have to possess more than a one-dimensional skill to remain in the discipline.

▶ HOSPITALS

Philosophy

The philosophy serving as a foundation for the hospital (as an institution in the health-care delivery system) is that wellness is a right, not just a privilege—that wellness is related to all aspects of a patient's life. Thus, health-care delivery should take a holistic approach in caring for the physical, emotional, social, and economic needs of the public.

Mission and Goals

The mission and goals of individual hospitals relate to the provision of inpatient, outpatient, comprehensive, and specialized health-care to the community or region. Related objectives address such areas as assuring quality control of health-care delivery, assuring continuing education for health workers, assuring quality control of equipment, and developing and communicating policies and procedures for institutional quality control.

Organization

The term *hospital industry* has become a common label for that part of the health-care delivery system where secondary and tertiary care are provided. We have come to expect a certain organizational structure in medium-sized and large business corporations, that is, a board of directors, a chief executive officer (CEO), a level of administrators reporting directly to the CEO, and succeeding levels of middle administrators, each reporting to the level above. At one of these levels in the individual enterprise, administrators are responsible for departments that do the company's business. Many individual hospitals today are owned by "giant" or major corporations; the organization of these companies is similar to that of corporations of comparable size. For the present discussion, however, we will consider organization only as it applies to the individual hospital.

Hospitals are headed by a board of directors or trustees. This board bears legal and moral responsibility for all hospital activities and has overarching responsibility for establishing hospital policy, distributing and safeguarding hospital assets, representing the public's interest, and approving medical-staff bylaws (which govern physician behavior in the hospital). The primary authority, acting at the direction of the governing board, is the hospital CEO, who is generally a president, although titles vary. A group of operational mangers report to the CEO. Collectively, hospital administration is responsible for the management of the hospital's financial, physical, and human, non-physician resources. There is also a chief of the medical staff, followed by chiefs of the various medical services offered in the hospital. The traditional services offered in most hospitals are medicine, surgery, pediatrics, obstetrics, psychiatry, orthopedics, radiology, and clinical laboratory; however, not all hospitals provide all services. Except for teaching hospitals, physicians are generally granted practice privileges but are not employees of the hospital. Figures 3-1 through 3-3 are examples of organizational charts for a 200-bed hospital, a 400-bed hospital, and a tertiary-care hospital respectively.

The traditional hospital discussed herein has already changed significantly with the introduction of a new movement in the health-

(text continues on p. 56.)

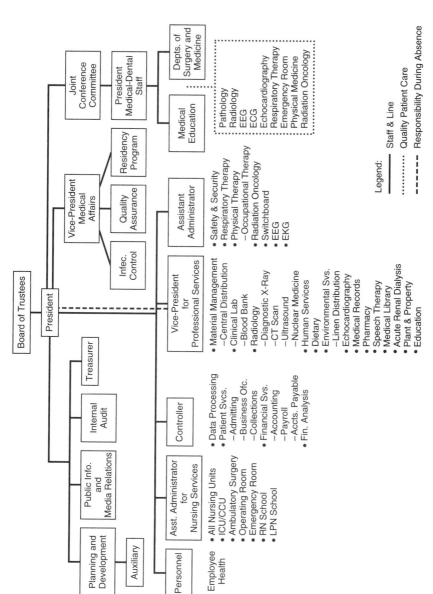

FIGURE 3-1. Organizational Chart of 200-Bed Hospital. [From *A Manual of Hospital Administration* (Vol. 1, p. 5:16), by H. S. Rowland and B. L. Rowland, 1992, Gaithersburg, MD, Aspen Publishers, Inc. Copyright 1986 by Aspen Publishers, Inc. Reprinted with permission.]

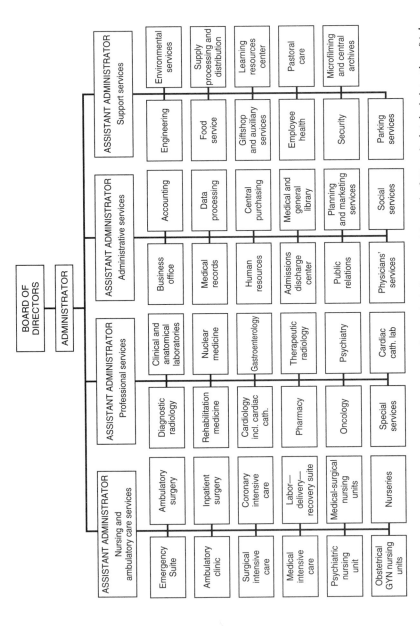

FIGURE 3-2. Organizational Chart of 400-Bed Hospital. [From *A Manual of Hospital Administration* (Vol. 1, p. 5:15)," by H. S. Rowland and B. L. Rowland, 1992, Gaithersburg, MD, Aspen Publishers, Inc. Copyright 1986 by Aspen Publishers, Inc. Reprinted with permission.]

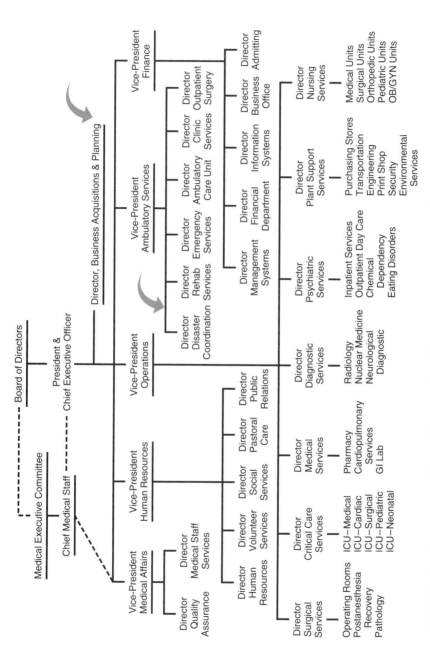

FIGURE 3-3. Organizational Chart of Tertiary-Care Hospital. [From *A Manual of Hospital Administration* (Vol. 1, p. 5:13)," by H. S. Rowland and B. L. Rowland, 1992, Gaithersburg, MD, Aspen Publishers, Inc. Copyright 1986 by Aspen Publishers, Inc. Reprinted with permission.]

care industry known as patient-centered care, patient-focused care, or patient plan of care. Although these terms express that same general concept, the latter term is actually defined as "a plan of care coordinated to include appropriate participation by each member of the health care team" [1]. Under such a plan, patients are placed in an area where a group of health-care professionals work as a team. They are cross-trained in fundamental medical techniques to assist each other so that patient's needs are met in a timely way and fewer persons are needed to do the work. Some basic types of medical care include those generally performed by nurses, laboratory technologists, respiratory therapists, and radiographers. State licensing, however, may limit cross-training of personnel from discipline to discipline. For example, because the application of medical radiation requires very specific knowledge, health professionals other than physicians and radiographers may be restricted from the use of radiation producing equipment in some states. Each discipline has its own specific knowledge base and it may be too ambitious to think cross-training can be accomplished expeditiously and economically in the depth needed for practice. However, the introduction of such movements is an indication of beginning efforts to reorganize health-care delivery as we know it today.

In this chapter we have looked at the health-care delivery system as a whole and how it has evolved. We have briefly touched on hospital organization. The next chapter will provide a detailed look at a radiology department in a contemporary hospital.

TEST QUESTIONS

1. The health-care delivery system includes the following professions/occupations:
   a. radiologic technologists only
   b. nurses only
   c. physicians only
   d. all of the above only
   e. all health-care delivery professions/occupations

2. Institutionalization of health care began in the United States in large hospitals. Match the following location with the appropriate well-known hospital.
   a. Cook County   1. New York
   b. Massachusetts General 2. Boston
   c. Bellevue   3. Chicago

3. Alternative forms of health care that may be recognized by some medical practitioners include:
   a. acupuncture
   b. herbal and homeopathic supplements
   c. vitamin and mineral supplements
   d. a and c only
   e. all of the above

4. The present health-care delivery system is identified as a three-tier level of care that includes primary care, secondary care, and superordinary care.
   a. true
   b. false

5. The American Medical Association (AMA), which began as a medical society, was established as the AMA in:
   a. 1800
   b. 1812
   c. 1847
   d. 1902

6. The most serious problem(s) in the practice of medicine during the Civil War was/were:
   a. lack of infection control
   b. lack of anesthetics

    c. lack of beds
    d. a and b
    e. none of the above

7. Some medical specialties began to emerge in large during the period of growth between:
    a. 1700–1750
    b. 1820–1860
    c. 1790–1799
    d. 1800–1805

8. Initial concerns of medical specialties practice, which fostered improved medical education and legislative regulation of medical practice, were focused primarily on:
    a. patient/physician relationships
    b. physician/physician relationships
    c. public image
    d. formation of the AMA

9. The practice of medicine prior to medical reforms in the early 1900s largely dealt with:
    a. epidemics
    b. infectious conditions
    c. lack of technology
    d. none of the above
    e. all of the above

10. The institution(s) that had the most profound effect on medical education reform was/were:
    a. Cook County
    b. Johns Hopkins Medical School
    c. The Carnegie Foundation through the Flexner Report
    d. Bellevue
    e. b and c

11. One of the most distinguishing elements of medical education at Johns Hopkins Medical School was:
    a. a clinical curriculum
    b. a school of allied health
    c. open admissions
    d. low tuition

12. Medical education reform began following an extensive review of medical schools and a subsequent report in:
    a. 1900
    b. 1910
    c. 1890
    d. 1935
    e. 1898

13. The first AMA Code of Ethics was adopted in:
    a. 1900
    b. 1847
    c. 1888
    d. 1900
    e. 1850

14. The concept of health insurance began in _____ as a social movement to guarantee an efficient and healthy worker population.
    a. 1900
    b. 1885
    c. 1955
    d. 1915
    e. 1945

15. Government health insurance stands as a landmark with the institutionalization in _____ of the Medicare and Medicaid entitlement programs.
    a. 1955
    b. 1971
    c. 1966
    d. 1988
    e. 1945

16. With the implementation of Medicare and Medicaid, health care began to be perceived by the public more as a right and less as a fee-for-service privilege.
    a. true
    b. false

17. Health-care planning began to achieve full stride in the _____ when programs such as HMOs and PPOs were developed.
    a. 1970s
    b. 1980s
    c. 1990s

    d. 1960s

    e. 1950s

18. Since the beginning of the _____ , health reform has been the most controversial agenda for both the federal and state governments.

    a. 1990s

    b. 1980s

    c. 1970s

    d. 1960s

    e. mid-1990s

19. The two most immediate crises for health care are access to health care and AIDS.

    a. true

    b. false

20. The concept of managed care began with businesses as early as the _____ following the intervention of government into health insurance:

    a. 1950s

    b. 1930s

    c. 1970s

    d. 1940s

    e. none of the above

21. Holistic health care is an approach based on meeting all persons' health needs and is focused on:

    a. emotional needs

    b. physical needs

    c. social needs

    d. economic needs

    e. all of the above

▶ REFERENCES

1. Anderson, KN, Anderson LE (Eds.) (1994). *Mosby's pocket dictionary of medicine, nursing, and allied health* (2nd ed.). St. Louis: The C.V. Mosby Company.

2. Anderson, OW (1985). *Health services in the United States: A growth enterprise since 1875*. Ann Arbor, MI: Health Administration Press.

3. Brown, R (1979). *Rockerfeller medicine men*. Berkeley, CA: University of California Press.

4. Flexner, A (1960). *Medical education in the United States and Canada: A report to the Carnegie Foundation for the advancement of teaching*. Washington, DC: Science and Health Publications, Inc. (Original work published by Carnegie Foundation, New York, 1910).

5. Glossary: Managed care terms. (1997) *Radiology Management 19*, (2), 7–8, 10–12.

6. Gregg, DW (1966). Managed care: Choosing an HMO. *Harvard Health Letter*, April (Special Supp), 9–12.

7. Institute of Medicine. (1988). *The future of public health*. Washington, DC: National Academy Press.

8. *Physicians and dentists directory: Indiana Kentucky*. (1904). Chicago, IL: Galen Bonsier and Co., Publishers.

9. Stevens, R (1971). *American medicine and the public interest*. New Haven, CT: Yale University Press.

10. McGregor, M (1989). Sounding board: Technology and the allocation of resources. *New England Journal of Medicine*, January 12, pp. 118–120.

11. Rayack, E (1967). *Professional power and American medicine: The economics of American Medical Association*. Cleveland, OH: The World Book Publishing Company.

12. Rowland, HS, Rowland, BL (1992). *Manual of hospital administration* (Vol. 1). Gaithersburg, MD: Aspen Publishers, Inc.

13. Starr, P (1982). *A social transformation of American medicine*. New York: Basic Books, Inc., Publishers.

14. Stevens, R (1971). *American medicine and the public interest*. New Haven, CT: Yale University Press.

15. Stevens, R (1989). *In sickness and in wealth*. New York: Basic Books, Inc., Publishers.

16. Williams, SJ, Torrens, PR (Eds.) (1988). *Introduction to health services* (3rd ed.). New York: John Wiley & Sons, Inc.

CHAPTER

4

The Evolution of the Hospital Radiology Department

► **OUTLINE**

- ► OBJECTIVES
- ► INTRODUCTION
- ► ORGANIZATION AND MANAGEMENT
- ► PERSONNEL POSITIONS AND RELATED WORK FLOW
- ► SERVICES
- ► RADIOLOGY IN TODAY'S HEALTH-CARE SYSTEM
- ► TEST QUESTIONS
- ► REFERENCES

▶ OBJECTIVES

At the conclusion of the learning opportunity the reader will be able to:

1. Describe basic differences between 1960s and 1990s radiology departments.
2. Identify and discuss the organizational structure of a 1990s radiology department in a 300-bed hospital and in an 800-bed hospital.
3. Describe the role of the department administrative director, the technical manager, and the technical supervisor(s) in a 300-bed hospital and in an 800-bed hospital.
4. Identify the various services (procedures) that may be offered in a 1990's radiology department and name the technical service personnel who perform the procedures.
5. Identify the high volume areas in a hospital other than the radiology department that may require that technologists be specifically assigned to them for radiology procedures coverage.
6. Explain how radiology is turning into a business and how changes that are occurring are affecting the practicing radiologic technologist.

▶ INTRODUCTION

The modern hospital radiology department is complex, highly technological, and very dynamic. The complexity of the department has brought about significant changes in staffing and departmental organization and management over the past thirty years. Some type of historical reference point is needed as background for discussion of the modern radiology department; for this chapter that reference will be events occurring in the early 1960s. This time period has been chosen for two reasons: (1) a number of readers probably can identify with this time period, and (2) the introduction of computer applications in radiology made a significant impact during these years. The most dynamic period of growth in radiologic sciences technology began in the 1960s.

It is important to note that the modern radiology department under consideration in this chapter is situated in a local hospital that has specialized equipment and laboratory facilities (secondary level of care), a large regional hospital that provides a specialized, highly technical level of health care (tertiary level of care), or a large, university-based (teaching) hospital (also tertiary level of care). The large regional hospital or university-based hospital will, of course, have a more complex organization and management structure and a greater number of state-of-the-art procedures available in the various departments.

A modern radiology department is diverse in imaging capabilities. X-ray is still the most widely used imaging modality and continues to be the bread and butter of radiology departments. Now, however, departments have other capabilities and/or specialty areas such as nuclear medicine, vascular/interventional technology, ultrasound, computed tomography (CT), and magnetic resonance imaging (MRI). Diversity in imaging capabilities, coupled with the fact that ultrasound and magnetic resonance do not use x or gamma rays to produce images, has resulted in many departments now referring to themselves as diagnostic imaging departments. Regardless of the name of the department, radiology remains an extremely important tool in the practice of medicine. In the following sections, we will look at today's radiology department from the perspective of organization and management, personnel, services, and the department's relationship to the health-care system.

▶ ORGANIZATION AND MANAGEMENT

In the early 1960s, organization and management of most radiology departments were rather simple and straightforward strategies. Figure 4-1 shows an organizational chart representative of a radiology department in a tertiary-care hospital (population of 500,000 or greater) at that time. During the ensuing years, the composition of radiology departments has changed to encompass new and expanding technologies and to meet the requirements of a far more complex health-care system. Figure 4-2 is an organizational chart that represents a contemporary radiology department in a community hospital (secondary level of care) or a small 300-bed tertiary-care hospital (tertiary care is generally thought of in terms of 400 to 800-bed facilities). Fig-ure 4-3 is an organizational chart of a modern radiology department in an 800-bed, university hospital. Although Figures 4-2 and 4-3 are representative of modern radiology departments, it is important to understand that there is a wide variation in the organizational structure of such departments from hospital to hospital. Community

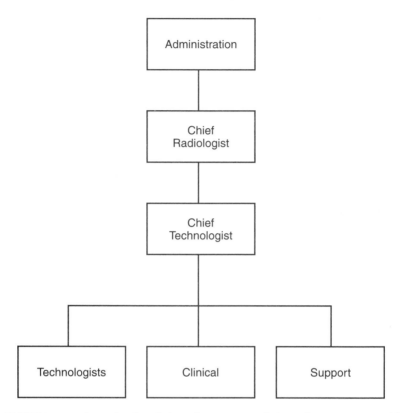

FIGURE 4-1. Organizational chart for 1960s radiology department. In this organizational plan, the chief technologist actually supervised technologists, clinical work flow, and support services.

hospitals are found in rural and suburban areas and most offer basic radiology services (i.e., orthopedic, chest, upper GI and colon studies). Tertiary-care hospitals generally offer the full range of diagnostic imaging technologies available at a given time. University hospitals differ from other tertiary-care hospitals because of the funded medical research that accompanies the academic component. Medical school faculty often have national or international reputations and the hospitals are in foremost or leading positions in the introduction of new techniques and new technologies.

The three organizational charts reveal a number of obvious differences: for example, the contemporary charts list positions that indicate an expansion in imaging modalities. A comparison of the charts

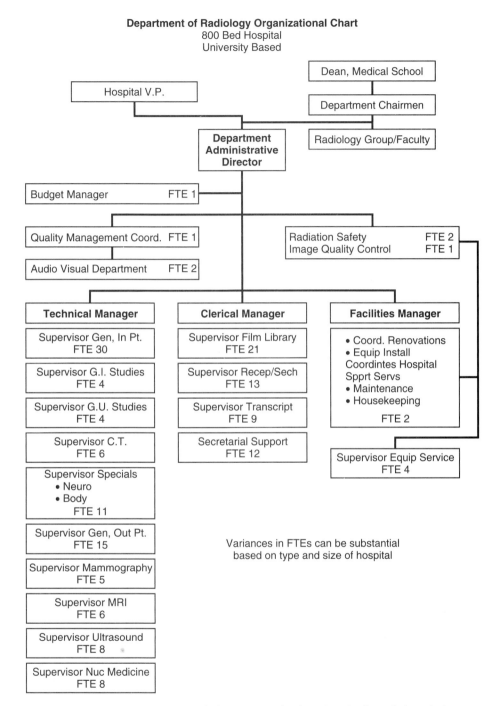

FIGURE 4-2. Organizational chart of 800-bed (university-based) hospital. [From *Introduction to Health Care Delivery and Radiology Administration* (p. 186) by S. S. Hiss, 1997, Philadelphia: W.B. Saunders Company. Copyright 1997 by W.B. Saunders Company. Reprinted with permission.]

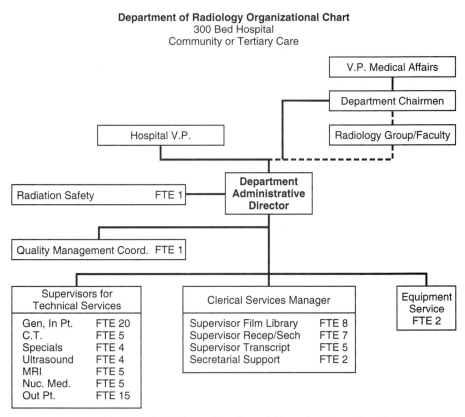

FIGURE 4-3. Organizational chart, modern 300-bed (community or tertiary-care) hospital. [From *Introduction to Health Care Delivery and Radiology Administration* (p. 187) by S.S. Hiss, 1997, Philadelphia: W.B. Saunders Company. Copyright 1997 by W.B. Saunders Company. Reprinted with permission.]

also illustrates how titles have changed. Other differences, which are not as apparent, will be discussed in the following section.

In the early 1960s, hospital radiologists sometimes shared in some expenses of the radiology department; medical supplies, film, and salaries are examples of such shared expenses. In addition to holding responsibilities as the department medical director, the chief radiologist, with some input from the chief technologist, often determined the needs for staffing and was primarily responsible for selec-

tion of equipment and persuading hospital administration to purchase it. Income for the radiologists was generally based on their
contract with the hospital; a percentage of the net revenues was paid
to the radiologists for their professional services. The radiologists
were members of the medical staff. Staff schedules, staff assignments,
and work flow were the responsibility of the chief technologist (at
the time, the highest ranking technologist in the department), who
also had input in selection of staff. A department might have two additional supervisory positions, one responsible for students and the
other responsible for the chief technologist's duties during that person's absences.

Today, the chief radiologist acts as the medical director of the
department, is very involoved in quality programs for the department
and the hospital, and works with other department and hospital personnel in a team approach to the purchase of equipment. He or she
is not responsible for hiring or firing staff but is often asked for input
when staff are evaluated.

Radiologists no longer share in any of the expenses of the department but may still be under contract to the hospital. Today, patients are billed directly for the professional services provided by radiologists. Radiologists may have other responsibilities assigned by
contract, and they serve as members of the medical staff.

Figures 4-2 and 4-3 illustrate the radiology department administrative director has oversight responsibilities for the same general
areas in the community/small tertiary and university hospital departments, that is, the position has responsibilities for departmental planning and organization, radiation safety, quality management, budget-
ing, staffing of technical and clerical services, facilities/equipment
maintenance. The individual holding the position is likely to participate in a team approach to selection of equipment, personnel evaluations, hiring and firing, policy and procedures, and productivity.
Both charts indicate that the administrative director reports to the
department's medical staff as well as to hospital administration (and
often to medical school administration in the case of the university-
based hospital).

In the early 1960s, the educational background required for the
department administrative director was that he or she be trained and
certified as an x-ray technician (now, specifically, radiographer). It
was also important that this person possess demonstrated supervisory skills, sound technical knowledge, and be well organized. In

most hospitals today, the department director is required to have a minimum of a bachelor's degree—and in many settings, a minimum of a master's degree—in addition to having completed training in radiologic technology. Some settings require that the department director have a master's degree but not necessarily education and training in radiologic technology.

Supervisors of technical services (other titles are also used) may report to the department administrative diretor and be responsible for the day-to-day operations (work flow) of the service (community or small tertiary hospital) or have the same responsibilities and report to a technical manager who has overall responsibility for the technical services (large tertiary or university-based hospital). Supervisory positions, which may or may not be lead positions, are generally responsible for day-to-day staffing and work flow for their respective imaging sections (lead position responsibilities involve active participation in imaging activities). Supervisors also participate in personnel evaluations and share in responsibility for quality control and improvement programs and equipment maintenance. Assigned duties for supervisory/lead positions vary from institution to institution depending upon the department size and whether the institution has a remote site (branch) imaging center.

The technical manager or technical supervisor is generally required to be certified in radiologic technology and in any related specialty area (i.e., nuclear medicine, MRI, mammography, etc). A minimum of a bachelor's degree and three to five years of supervisory experience may be required for this position; requirements vary to some extent according to the location of the hospital (metropolitan, urban, rural) and the pool of available health professionals.

The department administrative director, the technical manager, and the technical supervisors may have other duties delegated within the department or assigned by administration.

Many departments now have a business or budget manager—a position that is relatively new to radiology. This position typically holds or is delegated responsibilities related to clerical staff, payroll, support staff, and radiology nurses and may oversee the quality improvement program. Other responsibilities may include overseeing the orientation program for the department and the radiology information system. Many radiologist groups employ such a person to manage the business affairs of the group.

Business managers in radiology departments are generally required to have one to three years of supervisory experience with a minimum of a bachelor's degree; often, a master's degree is preferred.

▶ PERSONNEL POSITIONS AND RELATED WORK FLOW

In the early 1960s, radiology department personnel consisted of essentially those postitions shown on Figure 4-1. From the mid to late 1960s, nuclear medicine technologists were added to radiology department staff, and in the mid 1970s, ultrasound technologists were added. Many departments in the 1990s also include vascular/interventional technologists, mammography technologists, CT technologists, MRI technologists, radiology nurses, and a business manager. Many departments cross-train general radiographers in some of the specialty areas, for example, CT and/or MRI. It is evident that many different positions make up a modern radiology department; these positions include technical staff in each of the imaging sections of the department, clerical staff, radiology aides used as transporters and dark room technicians, and sometimes facilities management staff. In the following section, we will compare personnel in the two departmental organizational structures and describe various aspects of selected positions.

The technical supervisors (Figure 4-2) and technical service manager and modality supervisors (Figure 4-3) hold registries or certification in general radiography and/or specialty areas. Supervisory positions often require that the individual hold an associate or a baccalaureate degree (some require a master's degree); years of experience in the technical service is usually another criterion for supervisory positions.

The highest volume of procedures carried out in the modern radiology department, no matter how complex, is generated from inpatient and outpatient general radiography, including upper and lower gastrointestinal (GI) studies, genitourinary (GU) studies, chest films orthopedic films, and so forth. Note the number of full-time employees (FTEs) in Figures 4-2 and 4-3 in the general inpatient, outpatient, GI and GU studies categories and compare these numbers to the FTEs in the other categories. A radiology department in a 300-bed hospital may typically perform 100,000 procedures a year; in a larger tertiary care or university-based hospital up to 300,000 radiology exams may be performed [1, p. 186]. When the distribution of FTEs is considered in relation to the volume of exams performed, it becomes clear that x-ray is still the most widely used modality in the radiology department. Staff technologists may have attended community colleges, universities, hospital-based programs, or programs in trade/vocational-technical schools. Many states require that technologists be licensed; federal law (Consumer Patient Radiation Health and Safety Act of 1981) mandates that federal standards be set that states may use "for accrediting training programs and certifying individuals who engage in medical or dental radiography" [3, p. 294].

The radiology department may do a high volume of vascular/interventional procedures; if so, the technologists will have cross-training in this specialty. Such personnel, who fall under the category of "Specials" in the Figures 4-2 and 4-3, are required to maintain their radiologic technology skills and work in general radiography when not busy with vascular/interventional procedures.

Mammography and ultrasound are two more modalities housed in a many modern radiology department. Although the examples do not hold true from institution to institution, note that in our examples mammography has dedicated staff and a supervisor in the organizational structure of the larger, university-based hospital but not in the structure for the smaller hospital. Ultrasound has dedicated staff and a supervisor in both types of organizational structures; again, this may not be the case in all like institutions. All mammography technologists must be general radiologic technologists who have completed certification in mammography by the American Registry of Radiologic Technologists (ARRT). Ultrasound technologists have varied backgrounds with training in radiologic technology, nuclear medicine technology, nursing, ultrasound, other health-care programs unrelated to ultrasound, and/or even on-the-job training followed by certification.

Personnel in the nuclear medicine area in both the larger and smaller radiology departments shown in the contemporary organizational charts are made up of a supervisor and staff technologists. Education and training required for nuclear medicine technology have been discussed in an earlier chapter. Although nuclear medicine technologists in a radiology department may be cross-trained or be registered or certified in other modalities, most hospital positions require that they be registered or registry eligible because of federal and/or state standards relating to the use of radioactive elements or radiation in medicine or dentistry.

The MRI and CT services in the radiology departments shown in Figures 4-2 and 4-3 are similar in personnel structure to the nuclear medicine services. However, technical personnel in these services are generally radiographers who have advanced skill training in special procedures. Such personnel are considered to be cross-trained; some are cross-trained in both CT and MRI. In addition to clinical skills training, the advanced training most likely involves learning the principles of the special procedure, instruction in cross-sectional anatomy, and instruction in procedures specific to the modality.

Most technologists in a radiology department must cover in surgery; however, this area, with its high volume, may essentially become a specialty area. Consequently, several technologists may be assigned to work primarily in the surgery suites.

Another area that requires coverage and specifically assigned technologists is the emergency room x-ray suite. Several technologists are usually assigned in this area on the first shift. These technologists are often required to be cross-trained and perform duties in electrocardiography and phlebotomy in addition to their general duties as radiologic technologists. Radiographers on the second and third shift often are cross-trained and perform duties in CT scanning, electrocardiography, and phlebotomy in addition to their general duties as radioligic technologists.

Radiology departments have radiology nurses and radiology aides. Generally, the nurses and aides are supervised by the respective section supervisors (e.g., nuclear medicine, general radiography, etc.). The radiology nurses are responsible for monitoring patients who need close monitoring while in the department. They conduct nursing assessments and work-ups for patients who are getting vascular/interventional and other interventional procedures in x-ray, CT, ultrasound, and mammography. They assist with some of the stress cardiac studies done in nuclear medicine. Additionaly, radiology nurses may be responsible for providing some teaching, such as intravenous injection technique and CPR, to the staff. The supervisors and the nurses are responsible for developing and implementing all policies related to radiology nursing, infection control, and federal Occupational Safety and Health Administration (OSHA) regulations in the radiology department.

In the 1990's radiology department, aides often are required to be certified nursing assistants. They may be required to transport patients to different sections in the department, assist the nurses in patient monitoring and obtaining patient vital signs, assist in the dark room as needed, maintain the linen and transport equipment, assist in clerical areas if needed, and maintain the oxygen equipment.

Figures 4-2 and 4-3 show a single position, Clerical Services Manager or Clerical Manager, responsible for the four clerical components of the radiology department, with a supervisor and various numbers of FTEs making up each individual service—film library, patient reception/scheduling, transcription, secretarial support. Clerical duties are much the same today as they were in the early 1960s; there are, however, some variations. Modern hospitals may have centralized scheduling; if so, clerks do not have to be concerned with scheduling. They are responsible for registering patients, entering patient orders, communicating with the nursing units and physicians and their office staffs, and maintaining the patients' film files and reports. Some radiology departments (as in our examples) have their own transcription personnel whereas other departments may use centralized transcription services; in either circumstance clerical staff are responsible for mailing reports. Many modern radiology departments have added a radiology information system to computerize the department's clerical functions and patient tracking. In most hospitals clerical staff are required to have a minimum of a high school education; additional education or training, particularly with some computer skill, is preferred. It is also imperative that these personnel have excellent customer relations skills.

▶ SERVICES

The function of the radiology department is to offer a variety of procedures with a rapid turnaround in results. Radiology traditionally has provided service in nursing units, surgery, and the emergency room in addition to services within the department.

Services offered in the modern radiology department are reflected in advertisements appearing in news magazines and other such periodicals currently published for radiologic science professionals; in addition to radiologic technologist, advertised positions may include registered mammographer, ultrasound technologist, nuclear medicine technologist, CT and/or MRI technologist, cardio-vascular technologist, ultrasound cardiovascular technologist, echo-cardiographer, catherization lab technologist, special procedures technologist, and so forth. Thus, we can see that today's radiology department will generally include the following services: x-ray (including both radiographic and fluoroscopic examinations); vascular and interventional radiography; nuclear medicine; ultrasound; mammography; CT scanning; and magnetic resonance imaging. Brief definitions of these imaging modalities were provided in the first chapter and will not be elaborated upon here because discussion of the technological framework for the differing modalities is beyond the scope of this chapter.

Traditionally, other than for the services offered, radiology has essentially been a self-contained department without a great deal of interaction with other departments of the hospital. Today, radiology staff find themselves participating in cross-functional quality management teams and critical or clinical paths and as members of other committees within the hospital. Department personnel find that it is not unusual to have radiology equipment and services located in different areas of the hospital, such as digital fluoroscopy room located in the endoscopy suite, an interventional vascular suite located in surgery, a general radiographic suite in the emergency room, and a general radiographic room with chest unit in the outpatient pre-admission testing department. Some hospitals with patient-focused care units have radiology services on the nursing units. Many radiology departments today have nurses working in the unit.

▶ RADIOLOGY IN TODAY'S HEALTH-CARE SYSTEM

Regardless of all the changes that have occurred in the discipline and in the health care overall, radiology remains essentially a service or clinical support department in the health-care system. As health care continues to change, the radiology department must change as well, with more and more procedures occurring on an outpatient basis. Today's radiology department not only is in competition with radiology departments in other hospitals, but must also compete with free-standing radiology centers. There is great demand by physicians and patients for an efficient, speedy, and highly customer-oriented service. There is also great demand by these physicians and patients for radiology to provide a high quality service. Quality is also being scrutinized through government and accrediting agencies such as Joint Commission on Accreditation of Healthcare Organizations and the American College of Radiology.

Rising medical costs have brought about efforts to control escalation through health-care reform; reform is being pushed at all levels—public outcry; local, state, and national politicians; and, more recently, by the health-care industry itself. The industry has opted to react to the pressures being applied by becoming involved in the dialogue and attempting to have some impact in the decision-making process of the reform.

Health-care reform is having a noticeable impact on radiology already. Historically, the radiology department has been a revenue-producing department with a large operating budget. In today's health-care system, it is very probable that radiology and other revenue-producing departments will now be treated as cost centers rather than revenue centers. Peter Ogle, editor of *Diagnostic Imaging,* says, "Once a profession, Radiology is turning into a business. All of its costs are being ruthlessly examined" [2].

Changes that are occurring are having effects on the personnel in radiology departments. Health-care reform is causing a downward trend in patient days in the hospital and is impacting the number of procedures done in radiology. For a number of years, radiology departments have done cross-training resulting in the multicompetent radiologic technologist with training or specialization in more than one radiological modality. Today, radiologic technologists may be asked to cross-train in other disciplines to do such procedures as electrocardiograms, phlebotomy, electroencephalography, and some minor laboratory tests. This is particularly evident when technologists are taking positions in clinics and outpatient centers as well as in some hospital settings.

Many managed care programs have indicated that their process for selecting health-care providers/facilities will not be based upon cost alone, but also upon the quality care demonstrated by the facility. It currently appears that radiology will need to pursue outcome measurement for procedures to determine how the information provided impacted on the treatment of the patient.

In today's health-care setting, the demand for rapid turnaround for reports in radiology, lab results, cardiovascular results, and so forth is increasing. Even within the confines of the hospital, the pressure for rapid turnaround on reports and access to imaging is escalating. Today, many referring physicians demand the radiology report in 6 hours or less. Within the hospital they often require that images be accessible on the nursing units via electronic image management systems or that films be available for convenience of review and for discussion with the patient. Additionally, physicians may require that the films be sent to their office for review with the patient or that the physician be able to access the images via electronic imaging within his or her office. This type of demand has broadened the interest in electronic image management and computerized reporting that includes computerization of all medical records and computerized beside charting.

Most radiology departments today have become computerized in an effort to improve report turnabout times, and many departments are pursuing electronic image management systems to improve access to images as well. In this type of system, electronic images are expressed in digits for use by a computer. Such imaging systems should be capable of creating electronic images or digitizing hard copy images. One of the most commonly used systems is referred to by the term *picture archiving and communications system* (PACS). This system uses a local area network (LAN) for ease in image management and for transmission and archiving purposes.

Teleradiology is a type of telecommunication system, operated through a wide area network, which transfers digitized imaging studies outside a facility. In doing so teleradiology can extend radiology services to rural or remote areas that are unable to provide personnel with the appropriate expertise. That is, teleradiology permits radiology departments to communicate with distant offices, hospitals, and clinics that do not have a radiologist on site and thus leads to improved health-care services at such locations.

Although the technological explosion, triggered by the advent of the computer, brought many changes to radiology, other events have also had a dramatic effect on hospital and departmental operations—the introduction of medicare, diagnostic related groups, increased competition between hospitals, freestanding imaging centers, and competition from physicians who have elected to add imaging capabilities in their offices. Radiology departments are now involved in change that is being brought about by health-care reform. In many ways these changes will not be altogether new, because departments have already been cross-training technical staff, downsizing, and re-engineering concepts. However, for the first time, hospital radiology departments may be viewed as cost centers rather than revenue centers. It is anticipated that there will be more networking between hospitals, physicians, nursing homes, clinics, and providers in health-care delivery systems; there will be increased use of electronic image management over the next several years; there will be less money available for equipment and more exploration of innovative ways to prolong the life of current equipment.

Over the past thirty years, many changes in the radiology department have accompanied the explosion in technological advances. These changes tend to get a great deal of attention, and there is no doubt that these technological changes have added jobs to radiology departments and made the related work much more attractive as a career choice. These technological changes have also precipitated changes in radiologic technology educational programs to produce a more sophisticated, well-educated technologist.

TEST QUESTIONS

1. The most dynamic period of growth in technological applications in the radiologic sciences began in the _____ and continues today.
   a. 1980s
   b. 1960s
   c. 1970s
   d. 1990s

2. The organization of radiology departments in the 1960s was reflected in relatively simple organizational charts. This was because there were fewer modalities and most imaging procedures were contained within the department.
   a. true
   b. false

3. Many radiology departments have changed their names to Medical Imaging Department to reflect the procedures performed by the unit.
   a. true
   b. false

4. The most complex hospital organizational structure is found in a _____ facility.
   a. secondary level of care
   b. tertiary care
   c. neither of the above

5. Most modern hospitals require a minimum of a(n) _____ for administrative positions.
   a. certificate in a related discipline
   b. associate degree
   c. master's degree
   d. baccalaureate degree

6. The most widely used diagnostic imaging procedures are concerned with general inpatient and outpatient radiography.
   a. true
   b. false

7. The imaging modalities that became part of radiology departments during the 1970s were:
   a. mammography
   b. ultrasound

    c. nuclear medicine
    d. a and b
    e. b and c

8. In addition to the imaging specialties, large radiology departments often require that radiographers work on special assignment in areas outside the department. A good example of this need is:
    a. CT
    b. MRI
    c. surgery
    d. obstetrics/gynecology
    e. none of the above

9. Nurses who are employed by radiology departments may be responsible for duties associated with patient care such as:
    a. patient monitoring while in the department as needed
    b. patient assessment for various procedures
    c. work-ups for patients scheduled for vascular and other interventional procedures
    d. some teaching of patient care
    e. all of the above

10. Radiology procedures are provided in the radiology department only—both inpatients and outpatients are sent to the department. Therefore, there is no need to produce images anywhere else.
    a. true
    b. false

11. Which of the following radiology services may frequently be found outside the hospital in freestanding clinics or offices?
    a. radiographic/fluoroscopic services
    b. CT/MRI
    c. mammography
    d. a and b
    e. a, b, and c

12. Diagnostic imaging is conducted in other areas of the hospitals, such as nursing care areas and emergency rooms.
    a. true
    b. false

13. The impact of health-care reform on revenue producing radiology departments is that radiology procedures are becoming high cost areas.
    a. true
    b. false

14. Because health-care reform is resulting in downsizing of personnel, radiographers are being cross-trained in areas that may or may not have been available to them when in school prior to graduation. These areas may include:
    a. phlebotomy
    b. electrocardiography
    c. electroencephalography
    d. b and c only
    e. a, b, and c

15. All diagnostic imaging modalities must be viewed under the standards mandated by the Consumer Patient Radiation Health and Safety Act of 1981.
    a. true
    b. false

▶ REFERENCES

1. Hiss, SS (1997). *Introduction to health care delivery and radiology administration.* Philadelphia: W.B. Saunders Company.

2. Ogle, PL (1995). Trench warfare and the dean cat bounce. *Diagnostic Imaging, 17*(6), 5.

3. Stanfield, PS (1995). *Introduction to health professions* (2nd ed.). Boston: Jones and Bartlett Publishers, Inc.

UNIT

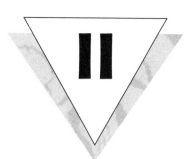

II

Introduction to the Practice of Radiography

CHAPTER

5

Radiation Protection

▶ OBJECTIVES

At the conclusion of the learning opportunity the reader will be able to:

1. Understand the biological basis of radiation protection.
2. Describe the units used to measure radiation.
3. Differentiate the various sources of radiation exposure.
4. Explain the ALARA concept.
5. Explain the principles of radiation safety.
6. Apply the techniques of radiation safety.

▶ INTRODUCTION

William Conrad Röntgen discovered x-rays in 1895. Soon after this discovery these seemingly marvelous rays were being put to use in the healing professions. However, it wasn't long before it was noted that excessive use of x-rays could cause hair loss and skin burns, not only in the patients, but also in the physicians and radiologic assistants. Within a few years, some of these people exposed to x-rays developed skin cancer, which eventually proved fatal. These were the some of the earliest known deleterious biological effects resulting from ionizing radiation. Ultimately it was realized that measures needed to be taken to prevent excessive exposure to radiation.

▶ RADIATION UNITS

In order to prevent excessive exposure it is necessary to be able to measure the amount of radiation to which an individual is exposed. For this reason physical amounts of radiation were quantified by a systematic set of units. Some of these units, developed in the 1920s and 1930s, are still in use today in the United States. However, the rest of the world uses a set of units called the International System of Units (S.I. Units), which are based on a simpler system of units.

Radiation is energy in transit, no matter whether the radiation is electromagnetic (x-rays or gamma rays) or particulate (alpha particles, beta particles, or neutrons). When an x-ray is absorbed in tissue it transfers energy to that tissue, where the energy can do work.

Some of this work can be used to break chemical bonds and thus cause damage to the cells that comprise the tissue. Thus it is important to be able to determine the amount of energy deposited in tissue. The original unit of radiation energy deposition was the *rad*, an acronym for *radiation absorbed dose*. This unit was defined as the absorption of 0.01 joule of energy in one kilogram of material. This unit has been replaced by the *gray*, which is the absorption of one joule per kilogram (1 J/kg). All of the radiation units are summarized in Table 5-1.

It is sometimes difficult to measure actual energy deposition in tissue. It is usually easier to determine the amount of radiation in a beam of x-rays. This is called radiation exposure. Radiation exposure is measured by the amount of ionization imparted to air. Air contains atoms and molecules that radiation can ionize by removing electrons. This electrical charge can be collected and measured, thus providing an estimate of the amount of energy transferred to the air by the radiation. The original unit of radiation exposure was the röntgen, defined as the production of 2.58×10^{-4} Coulombs of electrical charge to one kilogram of air. In S.I. units, the unit of radiation exposure has been simplified to one Coulomb per kilogram (1 C/kg).

Some types of ionizing radiation are more biologically damaging than x-rays or gamma rays. Generally, particulate radiations such as alpha particles and neutrons cause more biological damage than the electromagnetic radiations (x-rays and gamma rays) or beta particles, even when the same amount of energy is deposited in the tissue. For this reason a unit of radiation dose equivalent was developed. This unit was called the *rem*, an acronym for *röntgen equivalent man*. It represents the dose in rads multiplied times a quality factor. The quality factor is the increase in biological damage done by high en-

TABLE 5-1
Units Used in Radiologic Science

Quantity	Unit	Symbol	Traditional Unit	Symbol
Exposure	C/kg	C/kg	röntgen	R
Absorbed Dose	gray	Gy	rad	rad
Dose Equivalent	sievert	Sv	rem	rem

TABLE 5-2
Quality Factors [5]

Type of Radiation	Quality Factor (QF)
X, gamma, or beta radiation	1
Alpha particles, multiple-charged particles, and heavy particles	20
Neutrons	10
High-energy protons	10

ergy particulate radiations. Table 5-2 lists the quality factors for different types of ionizing radiations. For example, if a person receives an dose of 10 rads of neutrons, for which the quality factor is 10, this is equivalent to an exposure of 10×10 rads = 100 rads of x-rays, or 100 rems. The S.I. unit for radiation dose equivalent is the *sievert* and is defined as the dose in grays multiplied times the quality factor of the radiation. The sievert is the unit used for devising radiation protection standards. However, in the United States, all personnel film badge reports still use the rem, adjusted to thousandths of a rem (millirem, mrem).

▶ SOURCES OF HUMAN RADIATION EXPOSURE

Human exposure to ionizing radiation can never be eliminated entirely due to natural background radiation. Humans live in a sea of ionizing radiation from various sources. These sources may be natural, such as cosmic rays and terrestrial radioisotopes, or artificial, such as nuclear weapons fallout and industrial waste. Exposure from natural sources far outweighs any exposure from artificial sources. Among artificial sources of radiation exposure, medical use of x-rays is by far the most prevalent. Since we can control exposure of medical personnel and patients to x-rays, it is this exposure to which radiation protection efforts are primarily directed. Table 5-3 presents sources of background radiation in the United States to which everyone is exposed. Although human exposure to ionizing radiation will never be zero, it can be minimized through adequate environmental and radiological control.

TABLE 5-3
**Background Radiation Exposure
in the United States [1]**

Source	Annual Dose (mrem)
Natural	
Cosmic rays	50
Terrestrial radionuclides	80
Internal radionuclides	25
Artificial	
Nuclear fallout	1
Medical procedures	90
Man-made environmental	4
Total	250

▶ BIOLOGICAL CONCEPTS OF RADIATION PROTECTION

Ionizing radiation can cause definite deleterious overt and acute biological effects, such as skin erythema or epilation. Contemporary radiation protection standards are concerned less with such overt biophysical reactions and more with the effects of lower levels of radiation exposure. It is known that x-rays can cause cancer and genetic mutations. Radiation protection is primarily addressed to the idea that radiation exposure to workers and patients should be kept at levels that will minimize these carcinogenic or genetic effects.

It is well known that radiation will induce in reproductive cells mutations that will be passed on to future generations. Studies have shown that radiation-induced mutations can be harmful and that any dose of radiation, however small, to reproductive cells, may result in some genetic risk. Therefore, radiation protection standards and procedures have been developed to protect the reproductive integrity of patients and radiation workers. However, the risk of genetic mutations from very low radiation exposures may be so low as to be negligible in a practical sense. One must remember that risk represents only a probability of a certain event occurring. There are some risks in life that are so low, such as being fatally injured by a meteorite strike, that these risks may be effectively ignored as far as affecting the course of one's life. Many low-level radiation risks fall in this extremely low probability category.

Somatic effects of radiation, that is, effects that may result in the development of cataracts or cancerous malignancies, are also a concern of radiation protection standards. Radiation is known to be able to cause cancer, even at very low radiation doses. Since lower radiation doses will result in fewer occurrences of cancer, the radiation protection goal is to keep radiation doses as low as possible. However, the actual risk of cancer, which may appear years or decades after the initial radiation exposure, is very low within the limits of radiation protection standards.

Because low-level radiation exposure, spread out over a period of years, has the potential to produce biological damage that may not be seen for years following the radiation exposure, radiation protection standards and radiation safety procedures have been developed in order to keep radiation exposures to patients and radiation workers as low as possible.

The situation of the pregnant radiation worker or the pregnant patient presents a special situation in radiation protection. In this case genetic and somatic effects in both the mother and the embryo-fetus must be considered. Because of varying sensitivities to radiation at different times in pregnancy, the stage of the pregnancy in the patient or radiation worker must be considered. The first trimester of pregnancy is the most radiation-sensitive period for development of embryo-fetal lethality, congenital abnormalities, malignancies, and genetic effects.

Radiation protection is not only concerned with protection of the radiation worker but the general public as well. A radiation worker accepts some risk from radiation exposure, whereas the non-occupationally exposed individual usually has no knowledge of risks nor the freedom to avoid such risks. Therefore, there are different radiation protection standards for the occupationally exposed individual versus the general public.

There is a definite risk of genetic mutation or cancerous malignancy resulting from exposures to low levels of ionizing radiation. However, this risk must be weighed against the benefit accruing to the patient. The concept of risk versus benefit is very important in medical procedures and is fundamental in developing standards of radiation protection. All things considered, radiological technology is a very safe occupation when compared to risks encountered in every-day life.

▶RADIATION PROTECTION STANDARDS

Because of the risk involved, radiation protection standards have been developed by scientists working with the federal government. These standards, expressed as allowable doses of radiation to which a radiation worker or member of the general public may be exposed, were developed by the National Council on Radiation Protection and Measurements (NCRP) and are embodied in the Federal Code (10 CFR 20).

Radiation protection standards are stated in terms of *effective dose equivalent* limits. The effective dose equivalent (EDE) is the dose of radiation to the whole body or specific organs and tissues that takes into account differing radiation sensitivities that can result in genetic mutations and carcinogenesis. The EDE is expressed in sieverts or rems. It is used to provide the guidelines for maximal permissible radiation exposure to radiation workers and the general public. The recommended limits for radiation exposure are summarized in Table 5-4.

Effective dose equivalent limits differ for radiation workers and the general population and are further modified by reference to specific organ or tissue exposures and embryo-fetus exposures. For occupational exposure the annual effective whole-body dose equivalent limit is 5 rem. The dose equivalent limit for the lens of the eye is 15 rem. For all other tissues and organs, including bone marrow, breast, lung gonads, skin, and extremities, it is 50 rem. These exposures do not include the use of medical x-rays when the radiation worker is a patient.

The age of the radiation worker is also a factor in exposure limitations. At one time, no one under 18 years of age was allowed to work with ionizing radiation. This has been modified so that for educational and training purposes radiation workers less than 18 years old are limited to an annual effective dose equivalent of 0.1 rem.

In addition to annual dose limitations, a cumulative or lifetime dose limitation must be observed. This limit is determined by the age of the radiation worker. The total allowable cumulative exposure is

---

TABLE 5-4

Summary of Radiation Protection Standards [5]

A. *Occupational Exposures (Annual)*	*rem*
1. Effective dose equivalent limit	5
2. Dose equivalent limits for tissues and organs	
a. Lens of eye	15
b. All others (e.g., red bone marrow, breast, lung, gonads, skin, and extremities)	50
3. Cumulative exposure	1 rem × age in years
B. *Public Exposures (Annual)*	
1. Continuous or frequent exposure	0.1
2. Infrequent exposure	0.5
3. Dose equivalent limits for lens of eye, skin, and extremities	5
C. *Education and Training Exposures (Annual)*	
1. Effective dose equivalent limit	0.1
2. Dose equivalent limit for lens of eye, skin, and extremities	5
D. *Embryo-Fetus Exposures*	
1. Total dose equivalent limit	0.5
2. Dose equivalent limit in one month	0.05
E. *Negligible Individual Risk Level (Annual)*	
1. Effective dose equivalent	1

---

the age, in years, of the worker multiplied by 1 rem. For example, a 30-year-old radiographer is allowed a cumulative exposure of 30 × 1 rem or 30 rem. If a 29-year-old radiation worker has accumulated a total dose of 27 rem, then that worker, in his or her thirtieth year, can only accumulate 3 rem, instead of the usual 5 rem limit.

Guidelines for exposure limitations for the general public set limits lower than those for radiation workers. The effective dose equivalent for continuous or frequent exposures is 0.1 rem and for infrequent exposures 0.5 rem. These exposures do not include the use of x-rays for medical purposes when a member of the general public is a patient.

Embryo-fetus exposures for the radiation worker are also considered separately. The total dose equivalent for the embryo-fetus is 0.5 rem and the dose equivalent level in a month is 0.05 rem.

▶ RADIATION PROTECTION PROCEDURES

Current radiation exposure procedures are based on the ALARA concept. ALARA is an acronym for <u>As</u> <u>Low</u> <u>As</u> <u>Reasonably</u> <u>Achievable</u>. This means that all radiation exposures to patients and personnel are to be kept as low as possible while still obtaining the accurate diagnostic information needed from the procedure. ALARA recognizes that there will always be some radiation exposure to patients involved in radiological procedures using ionizing radiation, but it also recognizes that these exposures can be minimized.

Radiation workers need not be exposed to radiation at all during most of their normal work. In the special procedures where workers are exposed, the ALARA concept requires that the workers still must perform their duties while keeping their exposure to a minimum. Therefore, ALARA espouses the principle that radiation exposures can be kept below the maximum allowable level if proper radiation safety procedures and adherence to maximal exposure limits are followed.

The methods used to keep radiation exposures within desirable limits are not difficult to understand and use. Three simple concepts are of cardinal importance in minimizing radiation exposure: time, distance, and shielding. By following these three cardinal principles one may reduce radiation risk. The cardinal principles of radiation protection are to keep the *time* of exposure as short as possible, stay at as far a *distance* from the source of radiation as possible, and use *shielding* to absorb the x-rays when possible.

Time

The radiographer should strive to keep the exposure time needed to take a radiograph as short as possible. The dose of radiation is directly related to the duration of the exposure. The longer the exposure time is, the greater the radiation dose is. If the exposure time is doubled from 0.1 seconds to 0.2 seconds, the amount of radiation reaching the patient is doubled and potential radiation exposure of patients and workers is potentially doubled.

Distance

The operator of the x-ray machine should stay as far away as practical from the radiation source. The distance from the radiation source is inversely related to the radiation exposure. The farther one is from the x-ray tube, the less the radiation dose is. More precisely, the radiation dose is inversely related to the square of the distance. If the distance of the radiographer from the x-ray tube is doubled, the radiation exposure of the radiographer is not simply halved, but it is reduced by one-fourth. If the distance of the radiographer from the x-ray tube is halved, the radiation exposure of the radiographer is increased by four times. If a radiographer has to be in a room where a radiographic examination is being conducted, the radiographer should stay as far away from the x-ray beam as possible. An example of this is seen in the use of a portable x-ray unit, such as may be used to obtain x-rays from nonambulatory patients who cannot be moved. Portable x-ray machines are provided with a six-foot cord on the exposure trigger, so the radiographer can take advantage of the distance principle of radiation protection by moving the entire cord length away from the patient. Obviously the use of distance to reduce radiation exposure has little applicability to patients.

Shielding

All solid materials will absorb x-rays to different extents. Generally speaking, the denser a material is, the more radiation it will absorb. This is why lead is often used to provide shielding from x-rays. A radiographer should always strive to provide some sort of gonadal shielding to patients who are of reproductive age or who are potentially reproductive, such as pediatric patients. This may be done by interposing material that will absorb x-rays between the radiation source and the patient. When performing extremity exams, a simple method of patient gonadal shielding is to drape a lead apron over the patient's lap and lower abdomen.

During normal radiographic procedures (except for portable x-ray examinations and fluoroscopy and related examinations) the radiographer should not be in the same room as the patient. However, some times it is necessary for someone to assist in holding the patient, especially in the case of children and infants. When human-assisted patient restraint is necessary, the radiographer should *never* hold the patient. The first choice for a person to hold a patient during an x-ray examination is a family member or friend accompanying the patient. The next choice should be hospital or clinic personnel who are not routinely exposed to x-rays, but the same non-radiologic personnel should not always do the holding. If human-assisted patient restraint is necessary, the person doing the holding should wear a lead apron and lead gloves. In addition, the person doing the holding should never be in direct line with the primary x-ray beam. Lead aprons do not stop all x-rays, but only 50 to 80 percent in routine use, depending on the thickness of the lead and the energy of the x-rays.

Certain materials, such as lead, leaded glass, or high-density concrete, are used in the construction of x-ray rooms to contain x-rays within the facility. Because of this, there is generally zero or minimal x-ray exposure outside of x-ray rooms, such as at the control panel. Therefore, it is not normally necessary to wear additional lead shielding outside of the x-ray room.

Personal shielding may be used with the pregnant patient or potentially pregnant patient if it is absolutely necessary to perform an x-ray examination. Besides the exposure guidelines outlined above, a lead apron or shield may be placed over the uterus or totally surrounding the pelvis. In general, radiation protection procedures for the pregnant patient conform to the ALARA concept. The guideline to follow is that all radiographic procedures be performed to keep the radiation exposure as low as is reasonably achievable.

If a pregnant radiation worker performs only routine diagnostic procedures (excluding portable x-ray examinations and fluoroscopy and related examinations), it is not necessary for her to wear lead aprons in the clinic. However, if it is necessary to assist in portable x-ray examinations and fluoroscopy, an apron that wraps completely around the body is recommended.

Obviously the patient will always receive some radiation exposure during a radiological procedure. The amount of radiation received by the patient will vary according to the examination being performed, the kVp, the mAs, and shielding, if any. There will also be variations due to efficiency of x-ray production and image receptor speed. Most routine radiographic procedures will expose the patient to one rem or less. A single chest x-ray film will expose the patient to approximately 10 to 15 millirem. Representative doses to the skin, marrow, and gonads may be estimated, however. These are presented in Table 5-5. The values in this table are only approximations, but they may be used for relative dose comparisons among various radiological examinations. Generally speaking, examinations that require large field sizes and multiple films in a series will give the highest patient exposures.

TABLE 5-5

Approximate Radiation Doses to the Patient from Various Radiological Procedures [2]

Examination	Technique (kVp/mAs)	Skin dose (mrad)	Marrow dose (mrad)	Gonadal dose (mrad)
Skull	76/50	200	10	<1
Chest	110/3	10	2	<1
Cervical Spine	70/40	150	10	<1
Lumbar Spine	72/60	300	60	225
Abdomen	74/60	400	30	125
Pelvis	70/50	150	20	150
Extremity	60/5	50	2	<1

Personnel Monitoring

In diagnostic radiology the exposure of radiation workers to ionizing radiation is usually monitored by personal film badges. There are other types of personal radiation monitors, but the film badge is the most widely used. Film badges consist of a small piece of photographic-type film, similar to radiographic film, sandwiched in a plastic holder that may be clipped to the wearer's clothing. It is recommended that a pregnant radiation worker wear two film badges: one being worn at all times on the abdomen and designated as a "baby badge," and another film badge worn normally elsewhere on the body.

If the badge is exposed to ionizing radiation the exposed film will exhibit darkening upon development, with the degree of darkening proportional to the exposure received by the badge. In addition, metal filters made of aluminum, copper, or lead in the badge allow estimation of the radiation energy. There are metal filters in the back and the front of the film badge holder. These filters are of different thickness to account for the attenuation of radiation through the wearer's body. For this reason film badges should be worn with the correct side to the front.

Where on the body the film badge is worn is often a matter of personal convenience; there are no definite federal regulations in this regard. However, it is recommended that the badge be clipped over a belt, shirt pocket, or collar, or some piece of clothing that is not normally removed. If a film badge is attached to an outer jacket or laboratory coat, it is too easy to remove that jacket with the film badge still attached. If a lead apron is worn, as in a fluoroscopy or portable procedure, then the personal monitor should be positioned on the collar above the protective apron.

Several advantages of film badges are that they are inexpensive, easy to handle, not difficult to process, and reasonably accurate. Disadvantages of film badge use are that they cannot be worn for long periods because of fogging caused by incidental background radiation exposure, and possible exposure by temperature and humidity. They should never be left in an enclosed car or other area where excessive temperatures may occur. In addition, film badges should never be laundered.

It should be noted that film badges are not capable of accurately measuring total exposures less than 10 mrem. Therefore, on film badge reports, if a person receives an exposure of less than 10 mrem, that exposure will be expressed as "less than minimally detectable."

Film badges are only used for the monitoring of radiation exposure when on the job. If a radiation worker needs to be exposed to radiation as a patient, then the film badge should not be worn.

No one should be unnecessarily exposed to ionizing radiation. Suitable attention to radiographic technique will prevent repeat examinations, which will increase patient and possibly personnel radiation exposure. In addition, ionizing radiation must not be used frivolously. It is intended only as an aid to diagnosis in medical situations where the benefit of the procedure outweighs the risk associated with the radiation. Humans should never be exposed to radiation for mere instructional purposes, such as in the use of students for positioning models.

Proper attention to the ALARA concept, the cardinal principles of time, distance, and shielding, and consistent personnel monitoring will ensure safe and efficient implementation of radiation protection procedures.

TEST QUESTIONS

1. The traditional radiation unit used to measure radiation exposure is the
   a. röntgen
   b. rad
   c. rem
   d. sievert

2. The traditional radiation unit used to measure radiation absorbed dose is the
   a. röntgen
   b. rad
   c. rem
   d. C/kg

3. The traditional radiation unit used to measure radiation exposure of personnel and which is used on film badge reports is the
   a. röntgen
   b. rad
   c. gray
   d. mrem

4. The average exposure to the patient from a single chest x-ray is
   a. 10 mrem
   b. 100 mrem
   c. 1000 mrem

5. Which of the following is the single largest source of human-made background radiation exposure?
   a. food substances
   b. cosmic rays
   c. watch dials
   d. medical radiation

6. Which of the following is the single largest source of natural background radiation exposure?
   a. food substances
   b. cosmic rays
   c. radon
   d. medical radiation

7. The annual recommended effective dose equivalent limit for occupational radiation exposure to the lens of the eye is
    a. 1 mSv (0.1 rem)
    b. 50 mSv (5 rem)
    c. 150 mSv (15 rem)
    d. 500 mSv (50 rem)

8. The annual recommended effective dose equivalent limit for whole-body occupational radiation exposure is
    a. 1 mSv (0.1 rem)
    b. 50 mSv (5 rem)
    c. 150 mSv (15 rem)
    d. 500 mSv (50 rem)

9. The annual recommended effective dose equivalent (EDE) limit for occupational radiation exposure to the red bone marrow or the skin is
    a. 1 mSv (0.1 rem)
    b. 50 mSv (5 rem)
    c. 150 mSv (15 rem)
    d. 500 mSv (50 rem)

10. On January 1, 1998 the cumulative life-time exposure of a 35-year-old radiation worker is 200 mSv (20 rems). What is the maximum permissible whole-body radiation exposure the worker can accumulate during the coming year?
    a. 1 mSv (0.1 rem)
    b. 50 mSv (5 rem)
    c. 150 mSv (15 rem)
    d. 350 mSv (35 rem)

11. The total recommended effective dose equivalent limit for embryo-fetus exposures is
    a. 0.5 mSv (0.05 rem)
    b. 1 mSv (0.1 rem)
    c. 5 mSv (0.5 rem)
    d. 50 mSv (5 rem)

12. The monthly recommended effective dose equivalent limit for embryo-fetus exposures is
    a. 0.5 mSv (0.05 rem)
    b. 1 mSv (0.1 rem)
    c. 5 mSv (0.5 rem)
    d. 50 mSv (5 rem)

13. Body film badges should always be worn
    1. on the front of the body
    2. with the front of the badge away from the body
    3. in the ankle area
       a. 1 and 2
       b. 1 and 3
       c. 2 and 3
       d. 1, 2, and 3

14. When a radiation worker is pregnant
    a. she should wear two film badges, one at the collar, and the other on the chest
    b. she should wear two film badges, one at the abdomen, and the other elsewhere on the body
    c. she does not need any radiation monitoring
    d. she must not do any radiographic procedures

15. The lowest amount of radiation that can be reliably detected by a film badge is
    a. 1 mrem
    b. 5 mrems
    c. 10 mrems
    d. 10 rems

16. Which of the following are cardinal principles of radiation protection?
    1. time
    2. distance
    3. shielding
       a. 1 and 2
       b. 1 and 3
       c. 2 and 3
       d. 1, 2, and 3

17. A radiographic exam exposes the patient to 50 mrem. If exposure time is doubled and all other factors remain the same, the new patient dose is
    a. 25 mrem
    b. 50 mrem
    c. 75 mrem
    d. 100 mrem

18. A radiographer is 1 meter away from a patient undergoing a radiological examination. At this location the radiographer receives 4 mrem exposure. If the radiographer moves to a location 2 meters from the patient, what is the radiographer's exposure?
    a. 8 mrem
    b. 4 mrem
    c. 2 mrem
    d. 1 mrem

19. Gonadal shielding of patients is recommended
    a. in all examinations
    b. in all examinations when the shielding will not interfere with diagnostic information
    c. only for pediatric patients
    d. only for patients of child-bearing age, regardless of gender

20. Film badges
    1. are only used for the monitoring of radiation exposure on the job
    2. should never be laundered
    3. are impervious to the effects of moisture and heat
        a. 1 and 2
        b. 1 and 3
        c. 2 and 3
        d. 1, 2, and 3

▶ REFERENCES

1. BEIR III Report. (1980). The *Effects on Populations of Exposures to Low Levels of Ionizing Radiation: 1980.* Washington, DC: National Academy of Sciences.

2. Bushong, SC (1993). *Radiologic science for technologists* (4th ed.). St. Louis: The C. V. Mosby Company.

3. Curry, TS, Dowdey, JE, Murray, RC (1990). *Christensen's introduction to the physics of diagnostic radiology.* Philadelphia: Lea and Febiger.

4. Hendee, WR (1992). *Medical Imaging Physics.* Chicago: Year Book Medical Publishers.

5. NCRP Report No. 91. (1987). *Recommendations on limits for exposure to ionizing radiation.* Bethesda, MD: National Council on Radiation Protection and Measurement.

6. Statkiewicz, MA, Ritenour, ER (1983). *Radiation protection for student radiographers.* St. Louis: The C. V. Mosby Company.

7. Turner, JE (1986). *Atoms, radiation, and radiation protection.* New York: Pergamon Press.

CHAPTER

6

Overview of Radiographic Exposures

▶ **OUTLINE**

▶ OBJECTIVES

At the conclusion of the learning opportunity the reader will be able to:

1. Describe x-rays.
2. Identify four basic exposure (technical) factors: milliamperage (mA), kilovoltage peak (kVp), time (seconds), and distance (SID).
3. Discuss the production of the four exposure factors and the related elements of exposure control.
4. Define recorded detail as it related to visual and geometric properties.
5. Identify the problems of size and shape distortion and motion as related to the geometric image.
6. Discuss briefly the elements of density, contrast, source-to-image distance (SID), and object-image distance (OID) as related to recorded detail.

▶ INTRODUCTION

This chapter will provide an overview of radiographic exposures (x-rays) and a brief definition of radiation and how it is used to produce images on film. Students will be provided with much greater detail in the areas of radiation physics and radiographic exposures (techniques of film evaluation) as they progress through their radiography program. Only the most important information on major topics will be included here as an introduction to complex material. It is interesting to note that the information provided in this chapter may be found in many radiology-related textbooks regardless of their publication date. Because the information is related to natural science, the facts remain relatively true. "Many of the questions on Sister Mary Beatric's (one of the first technicians to take the Registry examination) exam would be applicable today. A few examples include: 'In what way does x-ray energy differ from light energy?' (and) 'What is the difference between primary, secondary, and stray or indifferent radiation?'" [3].

▶ DEFINITION OF X-RAYS

As mentioned in the first chapter, Wilhelm Conrad Röntgen, a physicist, discovered x-rays on November 8, 1895, at Würzburg University in Germany. Dr. Röntgen was not looking for the phenomenon that he observed; rather, he was working with the flow of current through a vacuum Crookes tube (Figure 6-1 shows a modified Crookes tube). When current was passing through the tube, he observed a light (fluorescence) coming from a chemical, barium platinocyanide, coated on a piece of cardboard several feet across the room. Because it was not known what these new rays were, they were called x-rays (x for unknown).

Although the creation of x-rays is an extremely complex process, an understanding of only a small portion of the associated physical concepts is needed to understand x-ray production. X-rays have certain properties or specific characteristics [1, 2, 7]: They

▶ Are invisible, silent, and cannot be felt.
▶ Are a form of electromagnetic radiation and have a dual nature, both waves and particles.
▶ Cannot be focused by a lens.

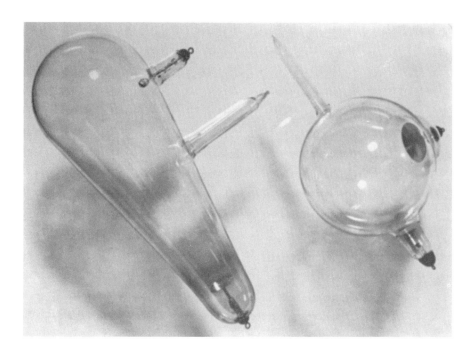

FIGURE 6-1. Left, simple x-ray tube with anti-cathode, modified from Crookes tube, from Röntgen collection. Right, simple cathode ray tube with plate cathode and rod anode, 1895. [From Klickstein HG. *Wilhelm Conrad Röntgen on a New Kind of Rays: A Bibliographical Study, Vol. 1. Mallinckrodt Classics of Radiology*, 1966.]

▶ Are electrically neutral.

▶ Travel in straight lines.

▶ Travel at the speed of light, 186,000 miles per second (3×10^8 m/sec) in a vacuum.

▶ Affect photographic film emulsion.

▶ Are heterogeneous and have a wide range of wavelengths and energy levels (a divergent beam of radiation is transmitted as photons—small bundles of energy—reach the x-ray film in varying degrees of energy, or wavelengths, to create an image; the variation in wavelengths is created as the electrons interact in different ways with the atoms of the target (Figure 6-2).

▶ Can convert to heat when passing through matter.

▶ Cause fluorescence of certain chemicals (i.e., crystals in screens).

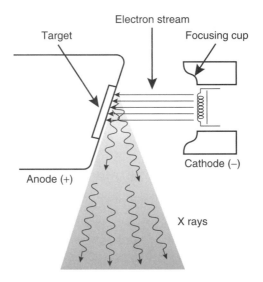

FIGURE 6-2.   Emission of electrons from the heated filament of the cathode. When free electrons strike the stationary target of the anode, x-radiation is produced at the actual focal spot of the anode. Rays of different wavelengths and penetrating power are produced, shown schematically as lower energy (longer wavelength) and higher energy (short wavelength) x-ray photons. [From Pizzutiello, MS, Cullinan, JE. *Introduction to Medical Radiographic Imaging.* Rochester, NY: Eastman Kodak, 1993.]

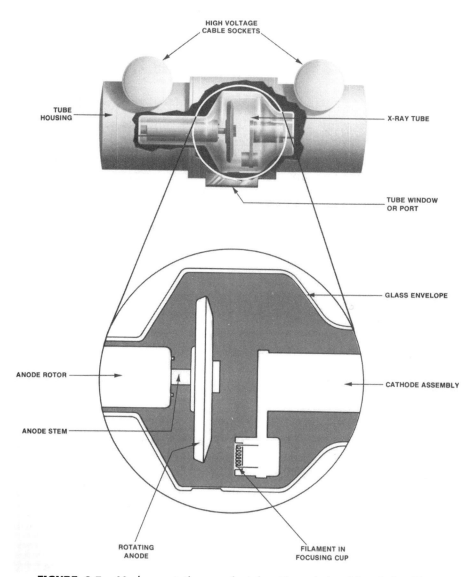

FIGURE 6-3. Modern rotating-anode tube. The relationship of the filament in a focusing cup (cathode) to the rotating anode is shown. [From Pizzutiello, MS, Cullinan, JE. *Introduction to Medical Radiographic Imaging.* Rochester, NY: Eastman Kodak, 1993.]

▶ Can ionize gases (ionization) through their ability to remove orbital electrons from atoms.

▶ Can produce biological changes in human tissue.

▶ Produce secondary and scattered radiation.

X-rays have no mass and therefore are not matter. In other words, we cannot see them because they do not occupy space in the visible world. X-rays are bundles of energy called photons (a quantum of electromagnetic energy). There are various forms of energy that perform work—for example, kinetic (motion), potential (position), chemical, thermal, electromagnetic, molecular, light, sound. "Changes in energy may be physical or chemical or both" [8].

Other than from material sources, radiation (x-rays) may be produced in an x-ray tube—that is how we are able to create images on film (Figure 6-3). X-ray tubes will be explained in more detail in specific materials on radiation physics and radiographic exposures as the student progresses through the radiography curriculum.

▶BASIC EXPOSURE FACTORS

There are four conditions that must prevail in a vacuum tube in order to produce x-rays [7].

1. Electrons must be set free. This is done by using 2 to 4 amperes to heat the tube so that it becomes incandescent. Some of the filament's electrons are freed and form a cloud (space charge) around the filament space. This is called thermionic emission (Figure 6-4).

2. The electrons must be focused. The electron stream is a narrowly focused beam that comes from the negatively charged focusing cup of the filament (cathode) and strikes a small spot on the target (anode). The narrowness of the beam depends on the size of the filament—the smaller the filament, the narrower the beam or line. This is called the *line focus principle* (Figure 6-5).

3. The electrons must be moved across the x-ray tube at a very high rate of speed from the negatively charged filament (cathode) to strike a highly positive charged target (anode)

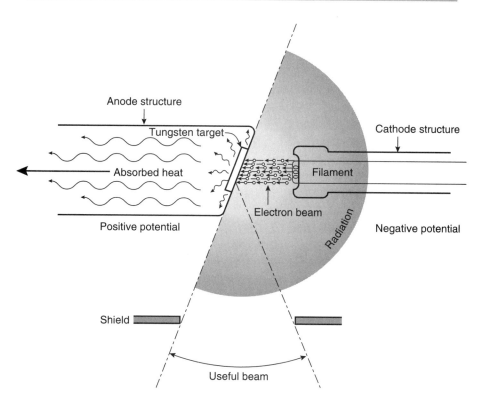

FIGURE 6-4. Thermionic emission. When a [tungsten] wire is heated to incandescence, an agitated unstable state is created in its atomic structure, resulting in emission of electrons from the wire's surface. These are loosely bound electrons from the outermost orbital electrons of the atoms of the metal (filament). Heating the metal causes sufficient energy to boil off the electrons and eject them from the filament. In reality less than 1% of the energy of this electron stream is used in the production of x-rays; the rest is converted into heat—heat that must be dissipated if the tube is to remain effective. [From Sante, LR, Fischer, HW (1962). *Manual of roentgenological technique* (20th ed.). Ann Arbor, MI: Edwards Brothers.]

(see Figure 6-2). The electron stream travels from negative to positive (cathode⁻ to anode⁺) at half the speed of light or more and produces variable wavelengths.

4. The electrons must be stopped suddenly. Fast moving (kinetic energy) electrons are stopped abruptly at the target (anode). This changes their energy to different forms, of which a small percentage is actually converted to x-rays.

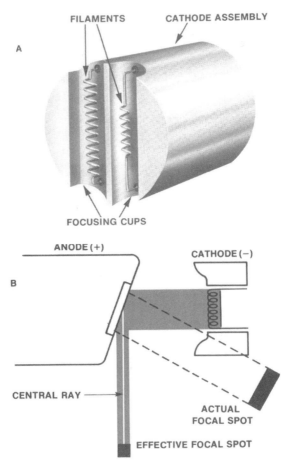

FIGURE 6-5. **a.** Cathode assembly showing focusing cups and two different-sized filaments. Their arrangements produce electron beams which are focused to narrow rectangles on the target. The smaller filament produces an electron stream of a small cross-sectional area and hence a smaller focal spot. **b.** Use of the line-focus principle and the angle of the target face (anode) to provide a small effective focal spot. When viewed from the direction of the central ray, the actual focal spot appears much smaller (effective focal spot). [From Pizzutiello, MS, Cullinan, JE. *Introduction to Medical Radiographic Imaging.* Rochester, NY: Eastman Kodak, 1993.]

The conditions presented above simply outline how x-rays are produced. Much more must be understood by radiographers, however, about the application of x-rays for medical purposes. Because this chapter is intended to present only introductory information, we will move on here to consider the basic exposure factors that are produced under the four cited conditions.

The factors referred to as milliamperage (mA) and kilovoltage peak (kVp) are the products that serve to create the latent image on the film. The image is called latent because the film must be put through chemical processing (just as ordinary photographic film) before the image becomes manifest or visible to the eye.

The mA is produced when the filament (cathode) is heated with electrical current and boils off electrons; this is how the electrons are counted in the flow of the electron stream (condition 1). The more the filament is heated, the greater the electron emission (thermionic emission), and the more electrons (and subsequent x-rays) are produced. Thus, milliamperage is what constitutes the amount or *quantity* of x-rays (radiation).

The kilovoltage is the force that moves the electrons across the tube (condition 2) and in modern equipment (other than single phase) operates at the highest levels of kilovoltage energy during an exposure. This highest level of kilovoltage is referred to as kilovoltage peak (kVp)—as seen in a waveform when it reaches its peak level. Just as we sometimes lose power in our homes during a storm, if for any reason we lose power to our x-ray machine, the peak level of kVp will drop and we will not get full exposure value; thus, the image on the film may be too light. However, this problem is rare in today's high technology radiology environment. Kilovoltage peak, then, constitutes the *quality* of the x-ray beam. This means that the higher the kVp, the more penetrating the beam of radiation becomes. This concept is complex and is presented only briefly here.

It is important to note the fact that kVp is more efficient at higher levels of energy. For example, 40 to 70 kVp is not as penetrating as is 80 to 100 kVp. Also, the level of kVp that is being used for any given set of exposures will not be affected by changes made in other exposure factors being used (e.g., mA). This means that kVp (e.g., 70 kVp) will retain its penetrating efficiency under all practical conditions associated with ordinary kVp settings for producing radiographic images in the clinical environment.

Two other factors play an important role in the effective outcome of the application of mA and kVp; they are *time* and *distance*. Time is a factor of duration. That is, the more time used with the mA, the more radiation is produced. Thus, the relationship between time and mA is proportionate; if you double the time, you will effectively double the quantity of radiation being produced. This proportionate effect may also be applied by doubling the mA. It is extremely important to remember this correlation because it has a direct relationship to radiation dosage. The combination of mA and time is called milliampere seconds, or mAs.

Kilovoltage peak is approximate and does not change in its effect by an increase in *time*. In other words, if you are using 80 kVp at .05 seconds, it will have the same effect at 1.0 seconds. This is not to say that the image will not be affected by other interactions.

Distance is a much more complex factor that affects the image outcome. Distance is a very important barrier used for radiation safety. The farther one is from the source of radiation, the less effect it has on human tissue. This is a cardinal rule of radiation protection. Radiation spreads out or attenuates as it travels away from the source; this phenomenon occurs because the greater the distance from the source, the more radiation spreads out and becomes less intense.

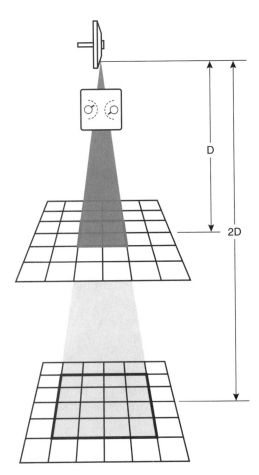

FIGURE 6-6. Inverse Square Law. Diagram showing how x-rays diverge and cover a larger area with diminishing intensity as they travel farther from their source. The intensity of radiation varies inversely as the square of the distance from the source. [From Pizzutiello, MS, Cullinan, JE. *Introduction to Medical Radiographic Imaging.* Rochester, NY: Eastman Kodak, 1993.]

In the application of medical radiation for diagnostic purposes, a standard distance, usually 40 inches, is used to produce most images of the human body. It is important that the source-to-image distance (SID) from the x-ray tube (target) to the film be set at the appropriate distance for each image; distance may vary with the type of image to be produced. If the distance is less than the standard 40 inches (e.g., 30 inches), the film will be overexposed; conversely, a distance of 80 inches would result in a greatly underexposed film. However, overexposure or underexposure will not occur in such circumstances if the quantity of mAs is compensated appropriately.

Distance obeys the inverse square law (Figure 6-6). This law states that the intensity of radiation is inversely proportional to the square of the distance. Notice how the image area is spread over a four times greater area by doubling the tube distance from the film surface. This causes the beam of radiation to become four times less effective as it was at the original distance. This must be compensated by adding four times more mAs quantity of radiation. On the other hand, for practical purposes the change in SID will not clinically affect the penetration ability of a given kVp setting.

Based on mAs (the combination of mA and time), the relationship between SID and mAs may be applied as follows. Suppose you already have a technique set up using 40 inches SID at 80 mAs and you wish to change the SID to 30 inches to reduce the mAs. In making this change you will need to calculate how much mAs will be required to maintain equal density in the radiographic image. Although there is more than one way to write the equation, the formula we will use for this example is:

$$\frac{\text{Old mAs}}{\text{New mAs}} = \frac{(\text{Original SID})^2}{(\text{New SID})^2}$$

$$\frac{80}{x} = \frac{40^2}{30^2}$$

$$\frac{80}{x} = \frac{1600}{900}$$

$$1600x = 72,000$$

$$x = 45 \text{ mAs}$$

This discussion regarding the four radiographic exposure factors is generally complex for most students. It does, however, become clarified with usage and is conceptually correct and very effective when the mathematical interactions are correctly understood and applied.

▶ RADIOGRAPHIC QUALITY

There are two areas of primary concern in radiographic quality (also known as definition): (1) visual elements and (2) geometric elements. Under these two areas are four sub-areas. Figure 6-7 provides a view of the sub-areas.

Visual Elements

Density and contrast comprise the visual elements of visibility of recorded detail and, again, may be likened to photography. If a picture of a person or thing appears too dark or too light, it is difficult to see detail. Remember that detail is information we want to see and that when the image is overexposed (too dark) or underexposed (too light), we will not see the information even though it may be there.

Density is the product of mAs (amount of electrons produced in the tube) and is represented by the amount of overall blackness seen in the radiographic image. The formula for density follows.

$$\text{Log} \ \frac{\text{incident of light intensity}}{\text{transmitted light intensity}} = \text{density}$$

This formula is complex and will be explained more fully in a course dealing with density and sensitometry.

Radiographic contrast is somewhat more complicated than density because it illustrates the differences between various thicknesses of anatomical structures as seen in the recorded image (i.e., bone, muscle, soft tissue). Contrast is based on shades of gray or tones produced by kilovoltage. The number of densities may appear in a range of lighter tones to darker tones (Figure 6-8). This is known as latitude. Two generally accepted radiographic scales of visible contrast are produced by different levels of kVp—the short scale and the long scale. The short scale, also known as high contrast, is represented by

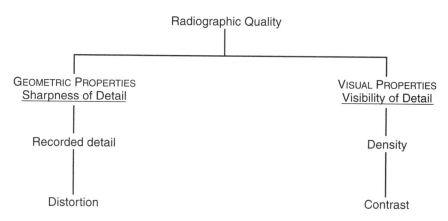

FIGURE 6-7. Sub-areas of radiographic quality.

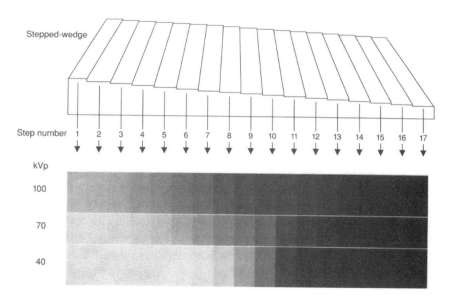

FIGURE 6-8. Latitude versus contrast. Latitude is related to the range of structures in a subject that can be imaged satisfactorily. In the strip labeled 100 kVp, more steps can be seen than in the strip labeled 40 kVp. Therefore, strip 100 has greater latitude than strip 40. Strip 100 also has lower radiographic contrast than strip 40. As contrast decreases, latitude increases, and vice versa. The difference in radiographic contrast between strip 40 and 100 could be the result of either a difference in subject contrast or a difference in film contrast. [From Pizzutiello, MS, Cullinan, JE. *Introduction to Medical Radiographic Imaging*. Rochester, NY: Eastman Kodak, 1993.]

a more black and white image. Fewer numbers of densities are seen in the radiographic image, so the range is short, with great differences from white to black and with fewer shades of gray. These short-range densities are produced at lower kVp levels (e.g., 40–70 kVp) as seen in Figure 6-8. As contrast decreases (with higher kVp), latitude increases; when contrast increases (with lower kVp), latitude decreases.

Long-scale contrast is represented by slight differences (lower contrast) in shades of gray and shows a larger number of densities as opposed to short scale's smaller number of densities. Long-scale contrast is produced at higher kVp levels, as seen in Figure 6-8 at the higher kVp of 100 and above. The important thing to remember about contrast is that it does not create recorded detail or information; it only enhances and therefore enables the viewer to better discern details.

There are two aspects of contrast—film contrast and subject contrast. Film contrast refers to the ability of the film to record various levels of density in the film emulsion. Like photographic film, radiographic film is manufactured with inherent contrast levels. Most people understand how to purchase photographic film (i.e., 400 speed, 200 speed, etc.). This type of speed relates to the ability of the film to respond to certain amounts of light (i.e., bright light, low light). Lower light requires faster film response.

Radiographic film speed also refers to response time to x-ray exposure. If a lot of x-ray is used, there will be increased response (if less x-ray is used, there will be decreased response). Response time is related to the type of film emulsion being used, which will be discussed fully in the sensitometric properties (or H & D curve) course dealing with film contrast, density, latitude, and speed.

Subject contrast pertains to the attenuation of radiation, or loss of photons, as the beam of radiation passes through the patient [7]. Because of the density differences in the anatomy, some structures are thicker than others; thus, they absorb more radiation and less radiation (fewer photons) reaches the film emulsion. This results in the formation of an aerial image (Figure 6-9) or an image outcome that depends on absorption and scattered radiation as it passes through bone, muscle, fat, and air. The radiation that exits the patient and reaches the film is called remnant radiation and may result in different contrast and latitude effects in the recorded image.

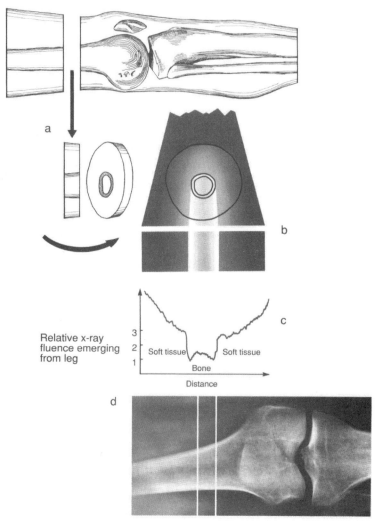

a

b

c

Relative x-ray
fluence emerging
from leg

3

2 Soft tissue

1

Bone

Soft tissue

Distance

d

FIGURE 6-9. Producing a radiography from exposure to processing. Multiple steps occur in the production of a radiograph beginning with exposure of the part under study. **a.** A transverse section of the distal femur is shown rotated to illustrate the absorption effects of the tissues of the lower thigh. **b.** The [anatomical] structures within the thigh cause a variation in the ... [flow] of the incident x-ray beam passes through the leg, the ... [flow] under the bone is ... [less] than that under the soft tissue because bone absorbs more x-radiation than the surrounding soft tissue. **c.** A graph is used to display the ... variations [in radiation] across the x-ray beam emerging from the thigh. The ... emerging [flow of radiation] from this soft tissue is three times greater than that from the bone. Therefore, the subject contrast between these structures is 3. **d.** The transverse section is displayed in the AP radiograph. [From Pizzutiello, MS, Cullinan, JE. *Introduction to Medical Radiographic Imaging.* Rochester, NY: Eastman Kodak, 1993.]

Geometric Elements

The geometric elements or geometry of the image relates to how clear or distinct the anatomy appears on the image—specifically, the quality of sharpness of the information of the anatomical structural lines or edges as seen in the radiographic image.

The elements of distance are source-image distance (SID), object-image distance (OID), and focal spot size (FSS). These factors are related to what is known as geometric blur. Also, distortion and motion must be eliminated from the radiographic image. Several terms are associated with a blurred image; such terms include *motion* and *unsharpness,* and some less frequently used terms, *penumbra* and *edge gradient.* Geometric blur, however, is initially the product of the FSS (small or large; Figure 6-10). When the smaller focal spot (filament) is used, the geometric blur, or structural unsharpness, is reduced.

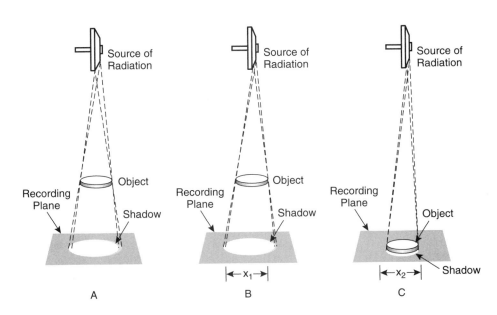

FIGURE 6-10. Geometry of image formation with the same SID. **a.** A large focal spot size with an increased OID, both of which increase image blur. **b.** A smaller focal spot size but still with increased OID and increased but improved image blur. **c.** A smaller focal spot size and reduced OID, which shows a superior result with minimal image blur. [From Pizzutiello, MS, Cullinan, JE. *Introduction to Medical Radiographic Imaging.* Rochester, NY: Eastman Kodak, 1993.]

SID is usually standardized at 40 inches. That is, the distance from the source (focal spot) to the image receptor (film) is maintained at 40 inches to produce most images. Generally, when the SID is maintained at a fixed distance, geometric blur is also minimized. This outcome is based on the concept of the line focus principle and also the heat capacity of the x-ray tube to be set at a certain distance from the film.

Heat is the main problem with x-ray tubes. Mostly what is generated in a tube when x-rays are created is heat. If the tube is far away from the part being examined, many more x-rays must be generated and thus more heat will be created within the tube. In order to reduce the blur, however, we want as much distance as possible without creating too much heat in the tube. Thus, a standard SID of 40 inches has been established as a compatible distance to minimize both heat in the tube and blur in the image. With the appropriate SID setting, geometric blur is reduced; magnification and size distortion of the image are reduced as well. As previously mentioned, SID obeys the inverse square law, which is extremely important to both the visibility and geometric properties of the image. Essentially, the greater the distance, the better the detail.

The object-image distance (OID) is an extremely important factor that affects geometric blur in the image. The object, or body part being examined, must always be placed as close to the film surface as possible. The less the distance between the film surface and the anatomy, the less the image is magnified or enlarged; that is, geometric blur is reduced (see Figures 6-10b and c). Generally, if there is an increase in the distance of the object from the film, there must be a compensatory increase in the SID to reduce the geometric blur that would be created by the increased distance between the object and film.

As previously stated, the focal spot size is related to the line focus principle. It is important to use the smaller size focal spot whenever practical to reduce image blur (Figures 6-10b and c).

Distortion involves the inaccurate representation of the size or shape of an anatomical structure as seen in the recorded detail of a radiographic image. Size distortion refers to magnification of the anatomy as opposed to its actual size. The anatomy being examined (e.g., hand, foot, chest) will appear unusually enlarged in the radiographic image if the anatomy is not placed appropriately close to the film (Figure 6-11). Shape distortion refers to elongated or

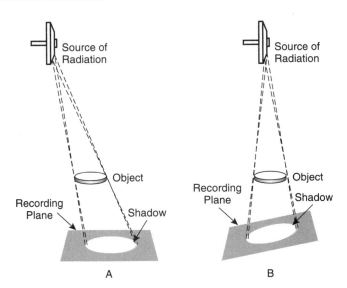

FIGURE 6-11. a. Distortion. Even though the source is not vertically above the circular objects, it casts a circular shadow, provided the object and recording plane [film] are parallel. **b.** Distortion. Distortion results when object and image receptor plane [film] are not parallel. [From Pizzu-tiello, MS, Cullinan, JE. *Introduction to Medical Radiographic Imaging.* Rochester, NY: Eastman Kodak, 1993.]

foreshortened shape of the radiographic image as opposed to the actual length of the anatomical structure (see Figure 6-11). This is the result of the object (anatomy) not being parallel with the film plane or the tube not being appropriately angled.

One other factor that must be discussed at this point is motion. Motion creates a geometric blur of the image—the anatomy becomes largely obscure to the viewer. One can relate to this type of problem when looking at photographs taken just at the moment the subject moved. Parts of the picture usually are blurred and related details are not well defined. In a radiographic image the same effect will occur if the patient moves during the exposure—the anatomical detail will be blurred. Therefore, the fastest exposure time that is compatible with the mAs, kVp, and SID setting should always be used to prevent the blurring effect of motion in the image. Additionally, whenever appropriate and possible, immobilization may be used to assist the patient in holding a fixed position.

The sum of all the image factors we have discussed plus the visibility and geometric properties result in the recorded image.

In this chapter we have briefly discussed basic exposure factors associated with radiographic quality as it relates to photographic or visual properties (density and contrast) and geometric properties (FSS, SID, OID, distortion, motion). The scope of radiographic exposures is sufficiently large that a specific course with laboratory experiments is generally included in a radiography program curriculum. Thus, this chapter has presented a broad overview of some of the most complex subject materials in image production. A detailed study of the factors and properties that affect radiographic exposures is required for the student to be able to apply this information in the clinical setting on actual patients.

TEST QUESTIONS

1. Which of the following statements is not characteristic of x-rays?
   a. X-rays are invisible, silent, and cannot be felt.
   b. X-rays travel in straight lines.
   c. X-rays are heterogeneous.
   d. X-rays are both waves and particles.
   e. X-rays can be focused with a lens.

2. X-rays have no mass and therefore are not matter.
   a. true
   b. false

3. The electron stream is a narrowly focused beam that comes from the _____ charged focusing cup of the filament of the tube.
   a. positively
   b. negatively

4. The latent image is created through the use of:
   a. kVp
   b. mA
   c. radiographic film
   d. a and b only
   e. a, b, and c

5. Kilovoltage is the force that moves electrons across the x-ray tube.
   a. true
   b. false

6. Kilovoltage peak (kVp) is more efficient at _____ levels of energy.
   a. lower
   b. higher

7. The effective outcome of the application of mA and kVp depends on:
   a. distance
   b. time
   c. focal spot size
   d. a and b
   e. a, b, and c

8. The factor that does not change in its effect with an increase in time is:
   a. milliamperage
   b. kilovoltage

9. For most diagnostic procedures, a standard distance of _____ is used to produce radiographic images.
   a. 72"
   b. 36"
   c. 40"
   d. 80"
   e. 45"

10. The inverse square law states that the intensity of radiation is inversely proportional to the square of the distance.
    a. true
    b. false

11. The exposure factors involved in the creation of the latent image include:
    a. mAs
    b. kVp
    c. time
    d. distance
    e. all of the above

12. Visibility of recorded detail involved the following elements:
    a. mAs
    b. contrast
    c. density
    d. b and c only
    e. a, b, and c

13. Contrast is primarily a function of tonal values produced in the application of:
    a. density
    b. mAs
    c. kVp
    d. none of the above
    e. all of the above

14. As contrast decreases with higher kVp, latitude increases.
    a. true
    b. false

15. Radiographic film speed refers to the response time of x-ray exposures to the type of film emulsion.
    a. true
    b. false

16. Some geometric elements that determine the sharpness of the recorded radiographic image include:
    a. SID
    b. OID
    c. FSS
    d. a and c only
    e. a, b, and c

17. The inherent problem associated with x-ray tubes is related to:
    a. heat
    b. age
    c. type
    d. none of the above
    e. all of the above

18. The recorded image is the result of a combination of visibility and geometric elements.
    a. true
    b. false

19. The radiation that exits the patient's anatomy and reaches the film is called:
    a. response effect
    b. aerial image
    c. remnant radiation
    d. none of the above
    e. a, b, and c

20. The most important thing to remember about contrast is that it creates recorded detail.
    a. true
    b. false

▶ REFERENCES

1. Carroll, QB (1993). *Fuch's radiographic exposure, processing and quality control.* Springfield, IL: Charles C Thomas.

2. Cullinan, AM (1987). *Producing quality radiographs.* Philadelphia: J.B. Lippincott.

3. Harris, EL. *The shadowmakers: a history of radiologic technology.* Albuquerque, NM: American Society of Radiologic Technologists, 1995.

4. Klickstein, HS (1966). *Wilhelm Conrad Röntgen, on a new kind of x-rays: Vol. 1. Mallinckrodt classics of radiology.* St. Louis: Mallinckrodt Chemical Works.

5. Pizzutiello, MS, Cullinan, JE (Eds.) (1993). *Introduction to medical radiographic imaging.* Rochester, NY: Eastman Kodak Company.

6. Sante, LR, Fischer, HW (1962). *Manual of roentgenological technique* (20th ed.). Ann Arbor, MI: Edwards Brothers.

7. Selman, J (1985). *The fundamentals of x-ray and radium physics.* Springfield, IL: Charles C Thomas.

8. Thomas, CL, Ed. (1993). *Taber's cyclopedic medical dictionary* (17th ed.). Philadelphia: F.A. Davis Company.

CHAPTER

7

Principles of Patient Care for Imaging Technologists

▶ **OUTLINE**

▶ OBJECTIVES

At the conclusion of the learning opportunity the reader will be able to:

1. Discuss basic assessment techniques.
2. Describe normal ranges for vital signs.
3. List principles of medication administration.
4. Define fundamentals of documentation techniques.
5. Demonstrate patient education methods.

▶ INTRODUCTION

Changes are occurring in the health-care industry that require non-physician members of the health-care team modify how they perceive the roles and responsibilities of their profession. Some of these changes relate to a concept commonly referred to as patient-centered care. Put into practice, patient-centered care requires that health-care professionals perform functions formerly considered not in their scope of practice. Whether this particular philosophy has been adopted in a hospital, professional expectations are requiring expanded bases of knowledge for those entering and new to the work force as well as for long-term members of the health professions.

The change in expectations is as true for radiologic technologists as it is for other professions. However, radiologic technologists may be better prepared than many other professionals for an expanded role; for example, radiographers may know more about general patient care than nurses know about x-ray production. Thus, response to change in the health-care environment may help decrease misconceptions about and enhance recognition of the professional role radiologic technologists have routinely performed.

This chapter will provide only a limited look at patient care; the area is so task- and skill-oriented that it requires detailed study and specific instruction in a number of techniques. Rather, the chapter is designed to be an introduction to patient care for imaging technologists, and the intent of the information is to help form a foundation on which technologists can begin the quest for knowledge. The student aspiring to be a true professional will seek to augment knowledge gained through classroom and clinical instruction and practice.

The content discussed in this chapter, when included in other publications, many times includes nursing care or nursing procedures terms. The goal of *all* health-care workers should be to provide quality care to the client by promoting, maintaining, and restoring a client's wellness [7]; nursing does not hold exclusivity on that particular concept.

The information provided on the following pages is related to *quality patient care*; all imaging technologists must be consciously aware of and adopt this concept for the knowledge to be useful and effective. The different territories and turfs of health care have become somewhat less concrete because of demands by the health-care industry for multicompetent and cross-trained workers. Rather than reducing responsibility, this blurring of traditional boundaries intensifies the need for each caregiver to know, observe, and/or apply the skills, processes, and procedures that constitute quality patient care.

Criteria for learning patient care, that is, learning objectives, are based in the cognitive, affective, and psychomotor domains. These domains are used in all areas and in all levels of education. Although explication of the separate domains can be quite complex, it can also be limited to very brief statements about each. Student technologists should think of these domains not only in relation to their own learning behaviors but also in terms of their role as patient care services provider. Simply stated, the cognitive domain "deals with the recall or recognition of knowledge and the development of intellectual abilities and skills" [1, p.7]; the affective domain "describe(s) changes in interest, attitudes, and values, and the development of appreciations and adequate adjustment" [1, p. 7]; and the psychomotor domain deals with "the manipulative or motor-skill area" [1, p. 7] and "acts requiring neuromuscular coordination" [4, p. 31]. Each domain breaks down into multiple categories of that particular classification scheme.

The technologist must be able to apply a broad knowledge base in providing proficient and skillful care to the individual client, significant others, and family [7]. In this chapter *client* will be used interchangeably with *patient*, although the term client implies viewing persons as consumers of health care and their health as a continuum that includes prevention of illness and maintenance of well-being as well as illness. In a society where terms used for traditional family relationships do not encompass the total reality of how people live and relate to each other, the term *significant other(s)* is being used to provide an inclusive designation for one person with an intimate or particularly close relationship with another.

The principal objective for any health professions student in learning patient care must be to obtain the knowledge and skills necessary to provide the patient with sensitive, safe, understanding, and proficient care. Although only a small portion of the basic patient-care skills technologists must possess to be competent practitioners in the professional role of radiographer will be discussed in this chapter, those examined represent broad and overarching areas of competence. Included are the skills of assessment techniques, vital sign analysis, data collection, general medication administration principles, documentation techniques, and patient education methods.

▶ ASSESSMENT

Assessment, by definition, is a process of systematically gathering, verifying, analyzing, and communicating data concerning a client [7]. The Principles of ARRT's Code of Ethics for the profession state in part: "The Radiologist Technologist assesses situations and acts as an agent through observation and communication to obtain pertinent information." A summary of the ASRT Position Statement for the radiographer includes the concepts that technologists should recognize patient conditions and provide for the physical and psychological needs of patients [8]. Assessment is an important and vital portion of the radiographer's professional responsibilities to patients.

Assessment of the client by the health-care provider begins in a problem-seeking direction [2]. The technologist should seek to obtain information from the client, significant other, or family that will assist the physician in making an accurate diagnosis. In order to acquire the data the technologist must demonstrate the ability to communicate with clients clearly, effectively, and therapeutically [3]. Details obtained from the patient can be classified in two categories: subjective and objective information.

Subjective information is data collected from the patient or other individuals accompanying the patient. Subjective data include statements the patient may make, such as "I have had pain in my back for three weeks." On many occasions the "I" statements made by the patient hold the key information for an adequate medical diagnosis.

Objective data are compiled from information the technologist acquires from observing, hearing, feeling, smelling, or from other validated resources, such as other health-care workers or the patient's medical record. An example of objective information might include that the patient has a productive cough upon deep inspiration. The assessment information should be pertinent to the complaint and the type of examination to be performed and documented in the patient's legal medical record.

Both subjective and objective data can be obtained from the patient or another source with the utilization of direct questions or open-ended questions. As the patient-technologist relationship develops, the patient will share increasingly appropriate information during the examination process. The technologist must listen to the information being provided by the patient and seek additional information to clarify any ambiguous or incomplete areas [8].

Information can be gathered from the client from the point of introduction. One of the first responsibilities of the technologist in gathering information is to determine the client's ability to communicate. This assessment should include both verbal and nonverbal communications. After the patient's identity has been established, the technologist must assess the patient's ability to understand the language and follow instructions and should inquire about any significant cultural and ethnical diversities. The technologist must also be alert to any developmental and spiritual differences in addition to any psychological or social considerations that may have significant bearing on how individuals should be approached as patients [8].

The basic skills of assessment for the technologist require very simple tools. Some of the instruments required are readily available. The tools include the human senses of seeing, hearing, smelling, and feeling in addition to the more traditional tools of assessment. The technologist should use the senses to assess the patient physically for normal and abnormal information.

The process of assessment should include visual inspection and olfactory (smelling) inspection; palpation of anatomical landmarks and body types to assist in the determination of size, shape, texture, and mobility of structures and masses; and evaluation of the extent of movement of bones and joints [2]. Percussion involves tapping of the body to determine position, size, and density of underlying structures as well as to detect fluid or air in a cavity. Auscultation (hearing) is the skill of listening to body sounds created by and in the lungs, heart, blood vessels, and abdominal viscera [7]. All together, these techniques are referred to as a physical assessment system. Technologists should use a systematic approach to analysis when performing an evaluation of a client's physical status.

Patients usually seen in the radiology department will present with a major complaint concerning their illness; sometimes this information may be provided by the referring physician, the patient, or a significant other. The complaint, in conjunction with supportive data from other health-care providers such as laboratory or physical therapy, should be documented and the radiologist informed of the findings.

▶ VITAL SIGNS

Vital signs, or cardinal signs of life, are indicators of a person's health status [7]. Vital signs include an assessment of pulse, respirations, blood pressure, and body temperature as a quick overview of the patient's physiological well-being. Although technologists may not obtain vital sign information on every patient, they must be skilled in the performance of related tasks in case the patient's condition requires such action. Baseline vital signs are essential on patients who are at risk for a change in health status, especially those patients involved with invasive procedures or contrast media administration. Technologists must consider factors that may alter or affect the normal ranges of vital signs for each individual patient.

Pulse is the blood flow through the body in a circuit creating a wave effect that can be detected in the peripheral arterial system by palpation [8]. Pulses can be palpated at areas where large arteries are close to the skin surface. Palpable pulses include the temporal, carotid, brachial, radial, femoral, popliteal, posterior tibial, dorsalis pedis, and apical. The tips of the middle three fingers of the technologist's hand or a stethoscope can be used as a tool in pulse assessment. The normal range for an adult pulse rate is 60 to 100 beats per minute; however, the technologist must be aware of and take any special or unique conditions of the patient into consideration if the pulse rate does not fall within the normal range, for example, a heart condition might cause a rapid pulse.

Respiration is the exchange of oxygen and carbon dioxide between the atmosphere and the cells of the body. There are two distinctive processes involved in respiration. Ventilation is the mechanical movement of the gases in and out of the body; breathing or perfusion is the exchange of gases at the cellular level. The technologist can only measure the ventilation aspect of respiration by specific assessment of the rate, depth, and rhythm of ventilatory movements [2]. The combination of an inspiration and an expiration constitutes one respiratory cycle. The respiratory rate should be calculated for one full minute with objective and descriptive characteristics observed.

Blood pressure is the force exerted by the blood against a vessel wall. This force is measured in millimeters of mercury (mmHg). Blood pressure measurements consist of the maximum (peak) force or systolic pressure and the minimum (trough) force or diastolic pressure as applied to the arterial wall at all times [7]. The average systolic pressure is 120 mmHg and average diastolic pressure is 80 mmHg in a healthy adult. A client's blood pressure can be measured using a sphygmomanometer (blood pressure cuff), auscultation (using a stethoscope), and palpation.

Body temperature is the physiological balance between the heat produced by the body and the heat lost by the body. Heat is produced in the body by a chemical process called metabolism. Body temperature can be measured utilizing a gauge called a thermometer. Three types of thermometers are available for measuring body temperature: mercury in glass, electronic, and disposable. Each of these devices has advantages and disadvantages, but most health-care institutions use electronic thermometers because of their accuracy and the reduced risk of cross-contamination between patients.

Three sites are used for measuring body temperature: the mouth, which is the most acceptable and convenient; the rectum, which should be used for infants and children and when the client is unable to use an oral thermometer; and the axilla, which is the safest but least accurate and the most time-consuming method. A temperature of 98.6°F or 36°C plus or minus one degree is considered the range of a normal temperature. Again, the technologist must remember that extrinsic factors can affect a patient's temperature, which may be outside "normal" ranges but still be within normal limits for that particular patient (see Table 7-1).

Vital signs vary for each individual patient. Assessment should include the variations of the normal ranges in the criteria established

TABLE 7-1
Vital Signs: Normal Ranges According to Age

Age	Resting Pulse Rate (beats/minute)	Ventilatory Rate (breaths/minute)	Systolic Blood Pressure	Diastolic Blood Pressure	Body Temperature
Newborn	120–170	30–50	80 ± 16	46 ± 16	96.6°F–98.0°F (A)
1 year	80–160	20–40	96 ± 30	66 ± 24	97.2°F–100.0°F (R)
3 years	80–130	20–30	100 ± 24	66 ± 22	99.0°F (R)
6 years	76–116	16–22	100 ± 14	56 ± 8	98.6°F (O)
8 years	70–110	16–22	104 ± 16	56 ± 8	98.6°F (O)
10 years	70–110	16–20	111 ± 16	58 ± 10	98.6°F (O)
16 years	60–100	16–20	118 ± 20	66 ± 10	98.2°F (O)
Adult	60–100	16–20	100–140	60–90	98.2°F (O)
Elderly	60–100	16–20	Maximum 160	60–90	96.8°F (O)

(A) = Axillary; (R) = Rectal; (O) = Oral.

by health-care institutions and the variations determined by factors affecting the individual patient, that is, sex, age, medications, and pathological conditions.

▶ MEDICATION ADMINISTRATION

The safe and accurate administration of medication is one of the technologist's most important responsibilities. The imaging professional must be knowledgeable about the policies and procedures of medication administration in the facility in which he or she practices. An understanding of any state or federal regulations and laws is essential prior to any administration of medication by technologists. Technologists should have an understanding of safe dosages, routes of administration, toxic reactions, side effects, adverse reactions, and indications and contraindications of use [8]. Before the utilization and administration of medication, the technologist must be familiar with pharmacological principles, including pharmacokinetics and pharmacodynamics.

Pharmacokinetics describes the interaction of drugs and body tissues. The interactions include reception, absorption, distribution, and metabolism of the drug and finally excretion of any byproducts of the medication. *Pharmacodynamics* is the study of changes in physiological functions of the body caused by drugs [5]. Effects of medication can include stimulating, slowing down, irritating, replacing, and weakening or killing cells.

Drugs are named by various methods. The chemical name of a drug consists of the exact chemical formula by which the drug is made. The generic name is the name by which the drug is labeled prior to its official approval for use. The trade name is the name used by the manufacturer as the marketing name for sale purposes [9]. Technologists administering drug therapy should be aware of both the trade and generic names of medications before administration. Drugs are classified by various methods. They can be categorized by their physiological effects on a particular body system or by their intended action.

Drug reactions vary from desired effects, expected side effects, toxic and idiosyncratic (unpredictable) effects, to allergic reactions. Reaction classifications can be mild, moderate, or severe, depending on the effects of the medication administered. Caution should be observed when the compatibility of mixing more than one medication is being considered. The imaging professional must observe for any unusual changes in the client's physical or emotional state, report such findings to the appropriate individual, and document the occurrence.

The route of administration depends on the drug's properties and the desired effect. The oral route is the easiest and the most commonly used method. Oral medications are slower in absorption and have a slower onset of action. Medications can be injected for quicker absorption by various methods, including subcutaneous, intramuscular, intradermal, and intravenous [5]. Topical medications are especially effective on mucous membranes and can be administered by direct application of the medication, inserting the drug into a body cavity, instillation or irrigation of fluid into a body cavity, or by inhalation. Radiopaque agents are considered diagnostic drugs, and technologists should follow all precautions in the administration of these agents. Observation of the Five Rights of Medication Administration [7] should be followed with the administration of every drug dose. These five rights are *The Right Patient*, *The Right Drug*, *The Right Route*, *The Right Amount*, *The Right Time*.

All drugs can both provide benefit or cause harm to a patient, according to their utilization. It should be the goal of all technologists engaged in the administration of medication to perform this skill in a safe, efficient, and effective method.

▶ DOCUMENTATION

The documentation of all care activity provided to a patient is required by many health-care accrediting agencies. This information should be contributed to and utilized by all members of the health-care team. Information such as who, what, when, where, how, and why concerning the patient's care must be included as part of the patient's permanent medical record. The five basic characteristics of reporting and recording patient care activities can ensure that communicated information is of high quality. These characteristics are accuracy, conciseness, thoroughness, currentness, and organization [7].

Information must be accurate! The imaging technologist must record only the factual information and must not include any personal opinion. Subjective data provided by the patient should be documented as such; information observed by the technologist should be noted as objective or interpretative data.

Any descriptive terms must be measurable using a standard system. For example, the meaning of a *large* cut or a *small amount* of blood will vary from individual to another; however, precise descriptions such as a 5-inch laceration or 300 cc of blood are clearly understood and do not require interpretation. Abbreviations used in the documentation of patient activity must include only those abbreviations approved by the institution. The technologist must be conscientious in assuring terms are correctly spelled and legible. The charting must be concise with short, easy-to-understand phrases using only key words and essential information. The record should demonstrate thoroughness and incorporate complete and relevant descriptive data [8]. Information must be current as it is documented. The longer the delay in making a patient activity entry, the more likely an error or omission will be made. All documentation entries must be dated, timed, and signed by the provider. Many institutions use military time to decrease the confusion of AM or PM.

An organized record contains documented information in a logical step-by-step format. Who it happened to, what happened, what happened as it happened, where it happened, and why it happened are documentation criteria for each technologist to consider as entries are made in the medical record.

All information concerning a patient must remain confidential. The medical record should be accessible only to those individuals with a need to know the information. Pertinent information relating to the procedure and/or the patient's condition must be available to the imaging technologists prior to the examination. Information relating to the procedure and or the patient's condition before, during, and following the procedure should also be documented in the medical record to ensure adequate continuity of care between all the health-care providers.

▶ PATIENT EDUCATION

Imaging technologists must assist patients and their families in understanding the activities of the imaging departments. Technologists are very knowledgeable and comfortable in a medical setting; however, many of the patients for whom services are provided do not comprehend the daily routines and activities of an imaging department. It is important to recognize that patients need assistance with understanding health-care situations and delivery methods, especially at a time when they may be frightened and under considerable duress about the state of their health. Although knowledge about the various classification categories of the cognitive, affective, and psychomotor domains can provide technologists with valuable background information in all the basic skills areas discussed in this chapter, it is particularly in areas such as patient education that this type of knowledge lends added depth to the technologist's ability to provide the patient and family members with information tailored to their unique characteristics.

It is important to point out that for the technologist, patient education should focus on areas pertinent to the examination, the equipment being used, possible side effects of medication administered, and any steps that should be taken after the examination to restore body systems to normal. Although patients may ask questions specifically related to diagnosis, treatment, and prognosis of a particular illness they fear (especially if the examination is symptom driven), answers to these types of questions do not fall within the scope of patient education provided by technologists.

Radiographers, as well as other health-care personnel, must utilize patient education as a tool in providing health care and explain to patients what outcome is expected of the relationship between the technologists and the patient [6]. Without attempting to diagnose, technologists should discuss in terms the client can understand the radiographic procedure and its purpose. Clients should be made comfortable and told approximately how long the procedure will take and what to expect during the procedure and after it is completed.

The process of teaching/learning often begins when the patient needs to know something or how to do something. Occasionally patients begin the learning process by asking questions (again, radiographers must be careful and answer questions only within their scope of practice). Caregivers must be proficient in helping patients to identify their needs [7]. Patient education involves assessing the needs of the patient, the family, and/or significant other.

Patient education assessment includes assessing not only needs but also willingness, readiness, and motivation to learn [6]. Basically, does the patient have any type of investment in the education process and how is the education going to be of benefit? The desired or expected outcome of the education must have a direct relationship to the patient and it must be of importance. The outcome objectives of patient education must be of mutual agreement between the patient and the care provider. If the patient has an outcome in mind different from that of the technologist, a common outcome from both parties is going to be difficult to obtain.

The learning abilities of the patient, family, and/or significant other must also be assessed. The educational background and comprehension ability are important assessment criteria. As mentioned previously, imaging technologists should provide the educational information in terms of the patient's understanding. It is important to remember that individuals learn in many different ways. Some learners are very visual and must see what they are being taught, some must hear and understand their instructions, while still others must involve the psychomotor aspects of learning. The technologist must be prepared to deliver the instructions; allow the patient, family, and/or significant other adequate time to internalize the information; and then assess for understanding.

Many times, when it is necessary to provide information regarding dietary considerations for a specific type of examination, instructions are given to the patient. Often, however, a spouse, significant other, or other type of caregiver will be responsible for food preparation and therefore should be included in any instruction of this type. Instructions following an examination are equally as important as those given prior to a procedure so the patient will know what to expect without apprehension. Technologists should provide instructions following an examination in a manner that will assist the patient to complete the requirements of the procedure in a safe, efficient, and effective manner and to the patient's satisfaction.

▶ CONCLUSION

This chapter began with a brief discussion of changes that are occurring in the health-care industry and the implications these changes may have for radiographers as well as other health professionals. As outlined in the objectives, the major focus of the chapter has been on establishing the principles of patient care for imaging technologists as well as establishing the concept of *quality* patient care. The chapter was designed with the purpose of providing not only basic information but also introducing ideas for students and instructors to pursue further in the classroom or for students to pursue on their own. It is assumed that a more comprehensive study of patient care will be provided for student radiographers in a separate course.

TEST QUESTIONS

1. The criteria for learning patient care are fundamentally based in the concept(s) of the:
   a. cognitive domain
   b. affective domain
   c. psychomotor domain
   d. all of the above
   e. none of the above

2. The affective domain is a very important area of behavioral learning. It is primarily reflected in the characteristics that include:
   a. motor skills
   b. intellectual abilities
   c. interest, attitudes, values
   d. a and c
   e. all of the above

3. Assessment techniques used to recognize a patient's condition and to obtain information regarding the radiographic examination of the patient include but may not be limited to:
   a. vital sign analysis
   b. documentation techniques
   c. patient education principles
   d. a and b only
   e. a, b, and c

4. Communication with patients must be conducted in such a way that the patient is responded to in a(n) _____ manner.
   a. clear
   b. effective
   c. therapeutic
   d. b and c
   e. a, b, and c

5. The statement, "I have had pain in my back for three weeks," is a(n) _____ type of statement.
   a. objective
   b. subjective

6. Observing, hearing, feeling, and smelling are _____ types of patient data.
   a. objective
   b. subjective

7. Match the sense/assessment technique in column A with the correct sense/assessment technique in column B.

   Column A
   a. smelling
   b. feeling
   c. percussion
   d. auscultation

   Column B
   1. tapping
   2. hearing
   3. palpation
   4. olfactory

8. One of the most important areas of patient assessment is vital signs. These include:
   a. body temperature
   b. blood pressure
   c. pulse and respiration
   d. b and c
   e. a, b, and c

9. Baseline vital signs are essential for patients at risk who are involved in invasive procedures with contrast media because:
   a. the patient's health status may change
   b. factors are present that may alter normal ranges of vital signs for each person
   c. vital signs are cardinal signs of life and are indicators of a person's health status.
   d. b and c
   e. a, b, and c

10. Match the vital sign in column A with the correct measurement in Column B.

    Column A
    a. pulse
    b. respiration
    c. ventilation

    d. blood pressure
    e. inspiration and expiration

    Column B
    1. one respiratory cycle
    2. blood flow
    3. exchange of oxygen/carbon dioxide
    4. systolic/diastolic
    5. mechanical movement of gases in and out of the body

11. Body temperature is the physiological balance between the heat pro-
    duced by the body and the heat lost by the body. Which of the following
    is correct?
    a. 98.6°F
    b. 36°C
    c. normal temperature range is within +1 or −1 degree and may vary
       with the patient's condition
    d. a and c
    e. a, b, and c

12. Gender, age, medications, and pathological conditions may all be factors
    that affect the individual patient with regard to patient assessment.
    a. true
    b. false

13. The radiographer must be familiar with _____ prior to utilization and
    administration of medications.
    a. pharmacological principles
    b. pharmacokinetics
    c. pharmacodynamics
    d. all of the above
    e. only two of the above

14. The interaction of drugs and body tissues include(s):
    1. reception
    2. absorption
    3. distribution
    4. metabolism of the drug
    5. excretion of byproducts
        a. 1 and 2
        b. 1, 2, and 3
        c. 1, 2, 3, and 4
        d. 1, 2, 3, 4, and 5

15. The interaction of drugs with body tissues is referred to as:
    a. pharmacological principles
    b. pharmacodynamics
    c. pharmacokinetics
    d. a and c
    e. a, b, and c

16. The study of changes in physiological functions of the body caused by drugs is referred to as:
    a. pharmacotherapy
    b. pharmacogenetics
    c. pharmacodiagnostics
    d. pharmacodynamics
    e. pharmacokinetics

17. Idiosyncratic effects of drugs are:
    a. desired effects
    b. expected side effects
    c. unpredictable effects
    d. a and b
    e. a, b, and d

18. Radiopaque agents are considered diagnostic drugs; therefore, all relevant precautions must be followed in the administration of these agents.
    a. true
    b. false

19. Patients' rights in administration of drugs into their body include the right:
    1. patient
    2. drug
    3. administration route
    4. amount of dosage
    5. time
        a. 1 and 2
        b. 1, 2, 3, and 4
        c. 1, 3, 4, and 5
        d. 1, 2, 3, 4, and 5

20. Information such as who, what, when, where, how, and why concerning the patient's care becomes part of the patient's permanent record.
    a. true
    b. false

21. The most important element(s) of communicated information include(s):
    a. accuracy and conciseness
    b. thoroughness and currentness
    c. organization

d. a and b

e. a, b, and c

22. Patient education for those undergoing radiological examination should be limited to:
    1. instructions pertinent to the examination
    2. the equipment being used
    3. possible side effects of administered diagnostic drugs
    4. possible diagnostic results
    5. post-examination instructions as appropriate
        a. 1 and 2
        b. 1, 3, and 4
        c. 1, 2, 3, and 5
        d. 1, 2, 3, 4, and 5

23. Without attempting to make a diagnosis, when providing health care, radiographers must explain the radiographic outcome of a procedure.
    a. true
    b. false

24. The outcome objectives of patient education must be of mutual agreement between the patient and the care provider.
    a. true
    b. false

25. Following radiographic examination, any necessary post-examination instructions must be communicated to the patient in a(n) _____ way.
    a. safe
    b. effective
    c. efficient
    d. all of the above
    e. none of the above

▶ REFERENCES

1. Bloom, BS (Ed.). (1956). *Taxonomy of educational objectives. The classification of educational goals. Handbook I: Cognitive domain.* New York: Longman.

2. Fuller, J, Schaller-Ayers, J (1990). *A nursing approach: Health assessment.* Philadelphia: Lippincott.

3. Harkness-Hood, G, Dincher, J (1992). *Total patient care. Foundations and practice of adult health nursing* (8th ed.). St. Louis: Mosby.

4. Harrow, AJ (1977). *A taxonomy of the psychomotor domain.* New York: David McKay Company.

5. Lehne, R (1990). *Pharmacology for nursing care.* Philadelphia: W. B. Saunders.

6. Redman, B (1993). *The process of patient education* (7th ed.). St. Louis: Mosby.

7. Potter, P, Perry, A (1991). *Concepts, process, and practice: Fundamentals of nursing.* St. Louis: Mosby.

8. Torres, L (1993). *Basic medical techniques and patient care for radiologic technologists* (4th ed.) Philadelphia: Lippincott.

9. Vocational Education Services, Instructional Support Division. (1991). *Medication Aide* [Curriculum]. Frankfort, KY: Cabinet for Workforce Development, Office of Technical Education.

UNIT

III

The Radiographic Environment and the Radiographer's Professional Role

CHAPTER

8

The Radiology Environment and the Radiographer

▶ OBJECTIVES

At the conclusion of the learning opportunity the reader will be able to:

1. Define the radiology environment.
2. Define and discuss work-related stress and stressors.
3. Explain the radiographer's control of his or her work environment.
4. Explain the concept of achieving the greatest good in the work environment.
5. Define moral responsibility and environmental ethics and discuss how they relate to radiologic technology.

▶ INTRODUCTION

Discussion in this chapter will focus on what actually constitutes the radiographer's work environment, what types of stressors are related to this type of workplace, ways in which radiographers can exert control over their role in the radiology work environment, and the role ethics plays in the successful adaptation of the radiographer to the work environment. In the author's view, this is one of the most pivotal chapters in the book because it is designed to strengthen the developing radiographer's understanding and belief in self as a responsible, competent, and ethical health professional.

It is important that radiographers know how to take charge of their own work environment. To accomplish this, radiographers need to be able to differentiate the elements of their particular professional role from those of other members of the radiology department, including the radiologist. The profession of radiographer requires that practitioners be technically competent, ethically competent, providers of patient-care services, advocates for radiation safety and protection, and users of initiative and independent judgment in applying radiologic techniques. Additionally, radiographers need to recognize that the manner in which they fulfill the responsibilities established by these elements determines in a large part how much control they have over their own work. Confidence in themselves as professionals and in their skills as well as knowledge about the work environment, their professional role, and certain principles, such as those originating in their professional codes of conduct, operate as enabling tools radiographers can use to exercise control in the work environment. It is hoped that emphasis on the radiographer's role in terms of the radiology environment will provide an accurate portrayal of radiologic technology as a full-fledged health-care profession.

▶ ENVIRONMENT

During the past two decades, the word *environment* has been used to encompass an extraordinary range of interests and issues and many times connote a global perspective. However, in the context of this chapter, environment essentially refers to two meanings: "circumstances or conditions that surround one; surroundings" and "the complex of social and cultural conditions affecting the nature of an individual or community" [1]. The intent of this chapter is to examine the role of the radiographer as it relates to the radiology environment.

One definition of *radiology* is "the branch of medicine concerned with radioactive substances, including x-rays, radioactive isotopes, and ionizing radiation, and the application of this information to prevention, diagnosis, and treatment of disease" [10, p. 1667]. The fourth chapter described several imaging modalities other than those just named that are components of modern hospital radiology departments. Thus, it is clear that the radiology environment is complex and includes many separate applications and responsibilities. Consequently, it is difficult to arrive at a simple description or definition of all the medical uses provided through the application of radiation and other imaging modalities.

The hospital radiology department is the work arena most common to the profession of radiologic technology. Regardless of where they are ultimately employed, almost all radiologic technologists learn their basic clinical skills in the hospital. Although the hospital is less frequently used today as an educational program base, many practicing radiographers attended hospital-based programs and thus gained both their didactic (academic) and clinical education in hospitals and their radiologic technology programs. Students who now acquire their didactic instruction in educational institutions still receive their clinical education principally in the hospital setting. Thus, the hospital radiology department constitutes the surroundings common to all radiologic technologists and is the foundation environment for the complex of social and cultural conditions affecting the nature of individual radiologic technologists and their common professional role. Additionally, although the hospital radiology department is separate from other departments, the radiographer must perform job duties in other areas of the hospital; thus, the radiology environment for radiologic technologists includes all surroundings where they perform radiographic procedures. Moreover, in the day-to-day performance of producing images, radiographers must be conscious of the artistic quality that their work reflects. Producing radiographic images is both an art and a science. No radiographer should present a radiologist or other physician with an image that is not of the highest quality. The radiographer controls his or her own work and should refrain from blaming poor films on patients and/or faulty equipment.

A high degree of stress may be associated with working in complex, high-technology environments. This is especially true when human illness is involved. The complex nature of radiology and the pressure to be accurate create such stress.

▶ WORK-RELATED STRESS

One of the first things that will become evident to students assigned to a hospital radiology department as they begin to learn clinical skills is the high stress level associated with this environment. The radiology environment is extremely dynamic, especially in facilities where a large volume of radiologic procedures are conducted, and often is very stressful. Radiologic technology is a patient-contact-oriented discipline; thus, there is reward in being able to help patients through direct contact. A high percentage of the radiographic procedures performed are time consuming and the pressure to perform accurately is often more intense than if the pace of work was slower. The volume and type of work and the degree of seriousness of a situation (i.e., emergency room, surgery, patient's condition) govern pressure. Other pressures associated with work-related problems may result from concerns about job security [10], work overload, lack of job content (limited variety of tasks), lack of control over own work, lack of support from supervisors, fellow workers, and sometimes from lack of understanding and support at home [12].

Concerns about job security may have been intensified for some persons by the 1990s' downsizing phenomenon and the trend towards patient-centered care. Other job security concerns may relate to role ambiguity, role conflict, and chronic stress/stressors. Role ambiguity may occur if an employee does not have a clear understanding of the job description for the position held or experiences a lack of recognition for performance in the position. If there is no mechanism in place for answering questions clearly or helping to solve problems, having to interact constantly with whoever is available rather than directly with a supervisor may cause frustration. Although documents relating to job descriptions and reporting lines exist in accredited hospitals, they may not necessarily be complied with fully or appropriately by those in leadership positions.

If parameters of job responsibilities are not clearly written and stated in terms understood by the personnel involved, employees sometimes assume duties outside their expected scope. Such individual behavior may create resentment or confusion among other staff members, and role conflict may result. Moreover, no matter how satisfied a person is with the type of work he or she does, the job environment may create stress. Stress is the body's nonspecific response to any demand.

> In health care, the term denotes the physical (gravity, mechanical force, pathogen, injury) and psychological (fear, anxiety, crisis, joy) forces that are experienced by individuals. It is generally believed that biological organisms require a certain amount of stress in order to maintain their well-being. However, when stress occurs in quantities that the system cannot handle it produces pathological changes. This biological concept of stress was developed by Hans Selye, who intended originally for stress to indicate cause rather than effect. But through a linguistic error, he gave the term stress to effect and later had to use the term stressor for cause [10, p. 1688].

In Selye's [9] own work, *Stress in Health and Disease*, he states, "Stress is associated with desirable or undesirable effects" (p. 15). In other words, stress is an outcome, not a cause; rather than different types of stress, there are different types of stressors or things that cause a biological response produced from within an organism (endogenous) or from outside an organ or part (exogenous). Stress, then, may arise from many nonspecific phenomena, such as emotional stress, stress of illness, stress of success, stress of failure, social stress, loss of sleep stress, and all such phenomena may be referred to as stressors.

Appelbaum [3] has discussed the impact of work-related stress on nurses and other health-care professionals. He identifies several considerations for the health-care manager regarding performance expectations (pp. 109–111). Some areas of concern (stressors) include lack of consistency between the job description and subsequent performance review; reward systems; coping with active illness, burnout, and cultural shock; and the turbulence associated with the realities of health care for sick and injured people.

The Flexner Report of 1910 [6] introduced a process into medical education that redirected the study of medicine from a largely art-oriented apprenticeship to a more biological sciences focus. However, according to Appelbaum [3], this Flexnerian model was not geared toward the social and psychological aspects of illness (pp. 143–144). Thus, naive health-care professionals have not been appropriately socialized for the realities of health care in a health-care setting. Appelbaum suggests some inservice activities to help newly employed nurses and other health professionals deal with stressful events. These activities may be conducted by health-care professional clinical supervisors and educators and include the following [3]:

▶ Development of a process for socializing new employees to avoid burnout and cultural shock when making the transition from the classroom to the intense real world.

▶ Use of a team approach in critical situations to minimize the burden of difficult tasks.

▶ Development of programs that emphasize interpersonal relationships and emotional outlets for appropriately dealing with acute illness and death.

▶ Use of inservice programs to develop multicultural awareness sensitivity.

▶ Initiation of more flexible and better balanced work schedules to reduce frustration.

The health-care environment is dynamic and constantly changing, and no specific health professional discipline experiences work-related stress more than another. Health-care delivery is a highly stressful type of work for all constituents. If workers do not understand their own role in the health-care environment, expectations related to emotional maturity may not be achievable and become unrealistic.

▶ CONTROL OF ENVIRONMENT

Obviously, there are factors in the work environment over which no individual employee has control. Therefore, when we discuss radiographers in terms of control of the radiology work environment, we are talking about radiographers taking charge of their own performance and conducting their work with confidence, knowledge, accuracy, and pleasantness. In order to attain such control, radiographers must know, respect, and comply with requirements not only for demonstrating the same moral behavior practiced by other health-care professionals but also for applying medical radiation safely.

When a person has the power of knowledge and is in control of a situation in which vulnerable people with illness are dependent on others to act ethically and perform their technical roles competently. The person with knowledge and control sets a climate of comfort and confidence for patients and other workers. This is true not only for the individual but for any group of people working together collectively as well. Similarly, any one person has the potential to create situations in which insecurity and apprehension impact patients and other workers. Lack of emotional control can act as one catalyst in establishing a negative climate.

Emotional Control

All professionals must be capable of maintaining emotional control over their own actions in the environment in which they work. One of the most important components of professional emotional maturity begins with understanding the moral principle of respect.

"In every action and every intention, in every goal and every means, treat every human being, yourself and others, with the respect befitting the dignity and worth of a person" [4, p. 50]. This statement infers that human beings are capable of making their own choices and therefore no value can be placed on their worth—they have infinite value. The concept of respect thus becomes even more important for those who are not, for whatever reason, capable of making their own decisions.

Beabout and Wennemann [4] propose that one criterion to determine whether you are treating another with respect is to consider whether your action is reversible; that is, would you want someone to do the same to you? Understanding the principle of respect clearly calls for a high level of maturity expected of professionals.

Beabout and Wennemann [4] further explain what it means to be a professional. They posit three ideas: (1) that one has a skill acquired through specialized training, (2) that one can give a rational account of one's own activities, explaining the "whys" and "hows" of one's area of expertise, and (3) that one is dedicated to using one's skills for the well-being of others (pp. 26–27). These ideas reflect a single ethic that transcends the particular profession; they also serve as the rationale for codes of ethics that deal with high ethical standards expected in professional behavior.

Pellegrino and Thomasma [8] have discussed professionalism in the context of describing medical virtues. In their definition of a virtue called *self-effacement*, they say:

> The term "character" may be taken in two ways. In a general sense, it summates the kind of person one is, as revealed by the virtues and vices one exhibits in one's attitudes and actions. More specifically, a person of character is one who can predictably be trusted to act well in most circumstances, to consider others in (his/)her decisions, to look at the long-term meanings of immediate impulses, and to order those impulses according to the canons of morality. . . . A person . . . (who) stands well with reference to the passions, who does not yield to extremes of self-interest, pleasure, or the desire for power (p. 146).

This latter summation of character, together with the concepts just set forth about respect and what it means to be a professional, establishes a framework for radiographers to develop emotional control in the work environment.

Safe Application of Medical Radiation

Pellegrino and Thomasma [8] also state,

> In a society such as ours, with its problems of poverty, homelessness, gaining access to health care, and denigration of the weak, we need to

maintain constant vigilance about protecting persons from undertreatment, abandonment, and inappropriate overtreatment. In both instances, we will be shepherding our technology to good human aims (pp. 124–125).

Although their discourse is physician-directed, this particular idea certainly applies to radiographers as well.

The most prudent way one can be protected from ionizing radiation is not to be within its vicinity of its travel. When it becomes necessary, however, that ionizing radiation be prescribed for application to human anatomy, the moral and legal responsibility for radiation protection is assigned to the person who applies the exposure—the radiographer or anyone who operates a medical x-ray machine. Chapter 5 has provided an overview on the nature of radiation and radiation protection standards. Accountability for radiation protection for patient, self, and others relates to several elements of the radiologic technologist's professional role.

The function of the radiographer is to produce radiographic images; this function has very little, if anything, to do with ordering examinations. The radiographer's education includes instruction in the best ways to minimize radiation exposure to patients, including the selective use of films, screens, processing, and maintenance of equipment. Even more important, with the exception of radiologists (physicians) and medical radiation physicists, the radiographer who is formally educated in an approved program receives more contact hours of radiation protection lecture than anyone else in medical practice. Moreover, equipment in today's sophisticated and computerized radiology environment is designed to eliminate many errors made by the "unwitting" radiographer or one who may have been poorly educated.

Consumer education would be well served if radiographers promoted their own profession through the dissemination of public information and education of the individual patient. Because there are unobservable risks inherent in the application of low-level medical radiation, clearly the value of the diagnostic benefits must be considered. The radiographer's responsibility toward the patient is carefully presented in several of the statements contained in the Code of Ethics (see statements 3, 5, 7, 8, and 9 in Box 8-1). Radiographers must fully exercise their knowledge and skills at all times to maintain quality imaging and prevent unnecessary repeat examinations. Ac-

---

BOX 8-1 Code of Ethics

1. The Radiologic Technologist conducts himself/herself in a professional manner, responds to patient needs and supports colleagues and associates in providing quality patient care.
2. The Radiologic Technologist acts to advance the principal objective of the profession to provide services to humanity with full respect for the dignity of mankind.
3. The Radiologic Technologist delivers patient care and service unrestricted by concerns of personal attributes or the nature of the disease or illness, and without discrimination, regardless of sex, race, creed, religion, or socioeconomic status.
4. The Radiologic Technologist practices technology founded upon theoretical knowledge and concepts, utilizes equipment and accessories consistent with the purpose for which they have been designed, and employs procedures and techniques appropriately.
5. The Radiologic Technologist assesses situations, exercises care, discretion and judgment, assumes responsibility for professional decisions, and acts in the best interest of the patient.
6. The Radiologic Technologist acts as an agent through observation and communication to obtain pertinent information for the physician to aid in the diagnosis and treatment management of the patient, and recognizes that interpretation and diagnosis are outside the scope of practice for the profession.
7. The Radiologic Technologist utilizes equipment and accessories, employs techniques and procedures, performs services in accordance with an accepted standard of practice, and demonstrates expertise in limiting the radiation exposure to the patient, self, and other members of the health-care team.
8. The Radiologic Technologist practices ethical conduct appropriate to the profession and protects the patient's right to quality radiologic technology care.
9. The Radiologic Technologist respects confidences entrusted in the course of professional practice, protects the patient's right to privacy, and reveals confidential information only as required by law or to protect the welfare of the individual or the community.
10. The Radiologic Technologist continually strives to improve knowledge and skills by participating in educational and professional activities, sharing knowledge with colleagues, and investigating new and innovative aspects of professional practice. One means available to improve knowledge and skills is through professional continuing education.

ceptable policy should include the right of the radiographer to question the need for certain films and, especially, repeat examinations; a second order for films might be an oversight (e.g., duplication of orders from consulting physicians). It is the radiographer's ethical duty to always act in the best interest of the patient.

Because of direct patient interaction, the radiographer, more than any other person, controls the activities in the radiology environment. Thus, quality radiography must be a constant concern.

One important concern is the application of patient immobilization. The practice of immobilization is completely at the discretion of the radiographer. Allowing the patient to be held by another person during radiation exposure has become disturbingly acceptable. Knowledgeable patient immobilization skills are still considered a proficient practice in patient-care management. Unfortunately, some radiology environments consider these skills useful only when they are absolutely unavoidable. Effective and skillful immobilization applied to a patient with whom one cannot communicate can avoid repeat radiographs that result in excess radiation dosage.

Children, for example, become angry and confused when physically restrained. However, unless a physical reason exists to not apply immobilization, children are not harmed when it is applied with expertise by a radiographer efficient in completing the task. The use of this safe and effective practice assists the parties involved in the procedure and others are not unnecessarily exposed to radiation while holding patients. For whatever reason(s), legal or otherwise, that immobilization is not being utilized by radiographers today, it is still a harmless, expedient, and frugal technique that tends to reduce repeat films, improve image quality, and achieve the greatest good.

▶ ENVIRONMENTAL ETHICS

Achieving the greatest good comes from an ethical concept that is reflected in the universal idea that we want to achieve the best outcome for as many people as possible. A number of related issues are being debated in today's health-care arena because the expanded knowledge base and advanced technologies that have provided state-of-the-art therapeutic possibilities and outcomes have also created problems related to access, rationing, the right to die, and so on. It may be more difficult now than it was in mid-century to validate what is meant by achieving the greatest good. Perhaps a good characterization is contained in a statement made by Pellegrino and Thomasma [8] in a discussion of fortitude: "medical fortitude . . . (is) the virtue that inspires confidence that physicians will resist the temptation to diminish the patient's good through their own fears or through social and bureaucratic pressure, and that they will use their time and training resourcefully to accomplish good in society" (114). This same thought can be related to achieving the greatest good and expanded to cover all health-care professionals. Clearly, this depends on (1) the degree of knowledge or expertise of the providers coupled with their enabling tools and (2) the magnitude of control such persons have over a particular situation.

The Radiographer and Achieving the Greatest Good

Knowledge and clinical skills are the enabling tools by which a radiographer achieves the greatest good for the consumer. He or she must demonstrate a clear understanding of the chain of variables in exposure factors and how techniques can be standardized for consistent quality.

Consistency in image quality is ascertained through careful daily attention to basic standards and values that apply to (1) equipment specifications (i.e., automatic exposure control), (2) exposure factors (i.e., mAs, kVp, time), (3) the careful application of both routine and special radiographic positions, (4) image quality critique criteria (i.e., image too light/too dark), and (5) film processing (i.e., chemistry temperature). Because of the many factors involved in the production of a radiograph, it must never be assumed that any single factor is as it should be unless it is checked prior to producing the radiographic image. In other words, a radiographer must have a systematic checklist (Figure 8-1) based on the above criteria.

A systematic approach provides a constant awareness that gives the radiographer the opportunity to use existing techniques or to quickly select alternative methods whenever routine techniques cannot be applied to specific disease or patient conditions (e.g., trauma). The radiographer must perform radiographic examinations as if each patient or client differs from the next, but the radiographer must

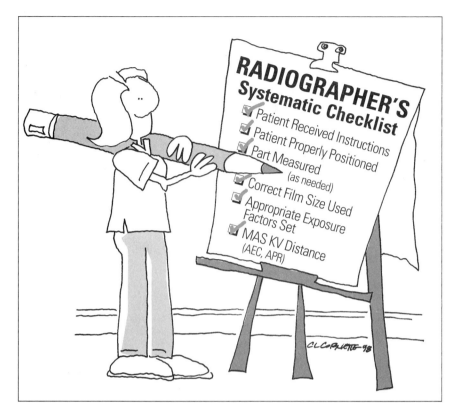

FIGURE 8-1. Radiographer's systematic checklist. (*Source:* Adapted by Carol Cornette.)

achieve the same image outcome. In other words, each radiographic examination has specific viewing parameters and image outcome (i.e., chest, pelvis, abdomen). When the radiographic examination does not involve an invasive-type procedure, the patient is in the immediate care of the radiographer only and, consequently, the radiographer becomes a decision maker and problem solver.

To illustrate a moderately complex situation where the radiographer must assume a decisive, critical-thinking, problem-solving role, let us consider the case of a patient in orthopedic traction who cannot be moved to the radiology department. The radiographer, therefore, takes a mobile radiographic unit to the patient. The patient's mending process will require that many radiographs be taken over several weeks. To eliminate repeats and to assure consistent image outcomes after an initial mobile radiographic examination has been completed, all exposure factors should be recorded on a card (including any unusual positions of the patient that might require an uncommon position of the machine and angle of the x-ray tube) and left with the patient's chart. This will communicate to the radiographer who will take that patient's next films what technique worked best and thus ensure accuracy of subsequent examinations.

Quality Improvement

Most radiology departments are accountable for doing at least an annual repeat rate analysis, which reflects an obvious concern for quality improvement and for reducing any excessive number of repeat examinations. Quality improvement is a very effective tool in maximizing environmental honesty and competence in the practice of radiologic technology. Over the past fifteen years quality improvement programs in the management of radiology environments have become critical, especially for hospital accreditation processes conducted by the Joint Commission on Accreditation of Healthcare Organizations (JCAHO). Quality improvement is synonymous with *continuous quality improvement* (CQI) and *total quality management* (TQM). These latter terms are used to reflect an approach to the continuous study and improvement of processes used to provide health-care services to meet the needs of patients and other recipients of health care [7, p. 181]. Two components are included in the overall concept related to quality: quality assurance and quality control.

Quality assurance is a program that includes appropriate individuals and groups or committees who are responsible for the structure and reporting of how quality is monitored [11]. *Quality control* refers to those aspects of quality assurance that deal with the technical procedures or the actual tests of imaging and processing equipment (Box 8-2). These tests are used to maintain daily consistency in radiographic procedure outcomes and to perform preventive maintenance. Such tests (e.g., of film processors and radiographic equipment) are conducted on regular schedules (i.e., daily, weekly, monthly, etc).

In recent years the revision and sophistication of automatic exposure controls (AECs) (sometimes incorrectly referred to as *photo-timing*) and automatic programmed radiography (APR) have opti-

---

BOX 8-2   Image Control Summary

Before Producing the Image:

1. Read the computer requisition or order on the patient to make sure that you are clear on what has been ordered and that all vital information has been included (name, social security number, age, history, etc.).
2. ALWAYS check machine to make sure that the tube is moved away from the table before bringing the patient into the room. This saves time.
3. Be sure that you can manage the situation alone. Experienced radiographers sometimes need assistance with complex or difficult examinations.
4. When taking the patient into the room, you should already have in mind exactly what you are going to do in the way of positioning, including any accessories you will require to complete the examination.
5. Exposure factors or techniques (including automatic) should be set after you have evaluated the patient's size, condition, and age and have generally observed the patient's behavior.
6. Although the processor should have been checked when operations began, check the processor periodically to assure that everything is okay (e.g., temperatures, chemistry, flow). This checkpoint is generally more important for processors where the workload is light; very busy radiology departments usually have someone overseeing this activity

After the Image Has Been Produced and Processed:

1. Assess the film for overall density and contrast levels (overexposures/underexposures/adequate exposure).
2. Assess the radiographic anatomy, that is, the part being examined and all articulating parts. For example, it is not sufficient to see the lungs only in a chest film, the areas just above the apices and just below the costophrenic angles must also be fully in view.
3. Assess the image positioning for corrections of angles and planes in relationship to the film plane (surface). Right angle views are generally required to provide depth in the anatomy (right angle refers to rotation from front to side).
4. Check the film markings *left/right* for accuracy. Also check all labels that include name and the number used to identify the patient's films. This is a must for any future legal purposes. A film without identification belongs to no one.
5. Always make a note for the radiologists of any unusual problems encountered in obtaining the films or anything unusual about the patient's anatomy that could be misleading in the image (e.g., skin markings that may be dense enough to show in the image).
6. Release the patient.
7. Always make sure the films are appropriately collected with the order and film folder.
8. Remember that you are the one who is responsible for the work you do in your work environment. You are the *only* one who controls what you do with your hands and your mind.

mized modern radiographic equipment techniques and have very much increased consistency in radiographic imaging. Simply stated, AECs act as the eye that sees radiation passing through a determined amount of human tissue; when enough radiation for a specific area of the body has penetrated, radiation production is automatically stopped. APR allows the radiographer to more readily select exposure factors for specific anatomical parts to be examined. These examples show how equipment can help provide consistent levels of density and contrast in the radiographic image when used properly. For example, given that radiographic images may not be photographically consistent 100 percent of the time, a consumer receives a chest examination and a follow-up examination is ordered six months or a year later. The radiographic images, if taken with the same machine and all other things being equal, should reflect a photographically equivalent outcome.

A major benefit in maintaining consistent levels of black and white in radiographic images is the increased probability of accurate interpretation of the images. Extreme differences in shades of black and white tend to obscure minute lines of information, that is, information among anatomical structures of equal and varying thickness. The imaging chain of any quality control program should include a well-organized monitoring system used to evaluate radiographic equipment and accessories; problems should at least be discovered during quality-control testing procedures, if not observed in the course of daily work.

The value judgment for film quality begins with the radiographer because he or she is the most knowledgeable about and aware of the technical variables and all the things that can go wrong when making a radiograph. Producing radiographic images is both an art and a science. The radiographer is the decision maker for all variables, including mAs, kVp, SID, patient position, and patient condition considerations. In other words, the image outcome depends almost entirely on the radiographer's knowledge and actions.

In achieving the greatest good, radiographers must not only become experts in the use and understanding of the technical tools of the profession, but also accept a moral responsibility for the patients they serve. The behavioral code of ethics for radiographers has already been discussed; however, moral responsibility is reflected in how individuals carry out their professional duties and how they respond to people.

Moral responsibility is very different from legal responsibility; that is, moral refers to some act we ought to do or that is nice to do whereas legal refers to some act the law states we must do. Moral and legal responsibility and accountability can become intermingled when an anomaly or an inappropriate behavior occurs. These occurrences may take the form of indifference, not caring, omission of duty, or not responding at all. This kind of moral responsibility permeates every aspect of our existence—personal and in the work-place.

In *Situation Ethics, the New Morality*, Fletcher [5] discusses the factor of response as the real key to responsibility: The essence of moral guilt lies in the failure or refusal to respond to the needs of others (p. 233), not in the failure to follow a rule or principle (p. 234). Fletcher notes that responsibility is too much thought of in a forensic way, meaning that there is too much argument about answerability to laws or rules rather than response to the calls and needs of people. Law attempts to prevent or limit freedom and openness and is thus designed to be impersonal and uniform (p. 235). By contrast, moral responsibility holds individuals accountable for their own behavior or actions, judgments, and decisions.

The preceding argument is not intended to be an all-inclusive discussion on moral responsibility but to point out that rules and laws are written in an attempt to prevent the most obvious or serious foreseeable problems, based upon what a reasonable person would do in given, similar circumstances. How people interact with other human beings and respond to their calls and needs depends on each individual's moral values (understanding of respect) and sense of human frailty. One place, outside the home, where moral response is critical is the work environment, especially in the helping professions. In the radiology environment, each radiologic technologist controls his or her work performance as an individual. True, there is work-related stress. However, even that type of influence must be placed in perspective with the whole schemata of why we are in a helping profession—to care for sick and injured people.

▶ CONCLUSION

The radiographer's responsibility in his or her own work environment has been identified. Some major responsibilities that have been discussed are understanding respect, moral responsibility, and enabling tools such as immobilization, basic standards and values, systematic monitoring, and a quality improvement program. Collectively, these responsibilities illustrate that the radiographer (practitioner) always has been in a position to function independently in his or her daily work and to control his or her performance and behavior. The radiographer has a critical responsibility in the application of medical radiation. The environmental ethics of the radiology department climate are established and controlled by those professionals who are in direct contact with patients and who possess the knowledge and skills to assure the highest quality of performance in radiographic examinations. The consumer has every right to expect professional, technical, and ethical competence from radiography practitioners.

The following position statement of the American College of Radiology (September 1980) expresses the recognition and responsibility of the radiographer.

> The Radiologic Technologist is qualified by education and the achievement of technical skills to provide patient care in diagnostic or therapeutic radiological modalities under the direction of radiologists. In the performance of their duties, the application of proper radiologic techniques and radiation protection measures involves both initiative and independent professional judgment by the Radiologic Technologist. Inasmuch as it is both desirable and necessary for all disciplines of Radiologic Technology to be recognized as professionals by government and other agencies, the American College of Radiology supports this position and recognizes the Radiologic Technologist as a professional member of the health care team.

TEST QUESTIONS

1. The professional role of radiographer requires that the individual radiographer be:
   1. technically competent
   2. ethically competent
   3. a patient-care provider
   4. a user of independent judgment
   5. an advocate of radiation safety and protection
      a. 1, 2
      b. 1, 2, 3
      c. 1, 2, 3, 4
      d. 1, 2, 3, 4, 5

2. The radiology environment is a complex branch of medicine that largely has its roots in:
   a. ionizing radiation
   b. radioactive isotopes
   c. x-rays
   d. all of the above
   e. two of the above

3. Stress is prevalent in almost all work environments. This is especially true in radiology primarily because of which factors:
   1. pressure to produce accurate images
   2. human illness
   3. limited contact with patients
   4. work conducted in a high-technology enviroment
      a. 1, 2
      b. 2, 3
      c. 1, 4
      d. 1, 2, 4
      e. 1, 2, 3, 4

4. Downsizing in the 1990s has created an increased level of concern related to _____ for many people working in health care.
   a. work overload
   b. job discontent
   c. job security
   d. none of the above
   e. all of the above

167

5. Role conflict sometimes occurs when there is poor communication involving:
   a. unclear job descriptions
   b. the lack of clear and understandable terms in job descriptions
   c. an employee assuming duties outside his or her scope of assignment
   d. b and c only
   e. a, b, and c

6. Work-related stress comes in a variety of forms. It may be physical or psychological and may be revealed in the body's nonspecific response to any demand. Such phenomena are called stressors and include:
   a. emotion
   b. illness
   c. failure
   d. success
   e. all of the above

7. One of the most important elements of coping with stress is to be well-informed of how to reduce stressors. Appelbaum has suggested some activities to help new health-care providers cope with transition into a new job. These include:
   1. socializing new employees to the real-world work environment
   2. using a team approach in minimize burden when appropriate
   3. using inservice activities for development
   4. providing flexible work schedules
      a. 1, 3
      b. 2, 3
      c. 1, 2, and 3
      d. 1, 2, 3, and 4

8. One very significant component of attaining/maintaining emotional maturity in the work environment is to:
   a. recognize the need for participating in inservice activities
   b. recognize the need for socializing
   c. recognize the need for participating in outside activities
   d. practice the concept of human respect
   e. none of the above

9. The radiographer is often not only the patient's most direct contact with medical radiology personnel but may be the patient's only contact. He

or she must therefore take full responsibiity for the appropriate application of _____.
a. quality improvement techniques
b. radiation protection techniques
c. image processing techniques
d. all of the above
e. none of the above

10. To avoid repeat films, one of the most effective techniques associated
with patient-care management is to apply:
a. methods of holding patients manually
b. limits on repeats
c. knowledgeable immobilization techniques
d. none of the above
e. all of the above

11. The concept of achieving the greatest good is based on the idea of:
a. the Golden Rule
b. patient dependence
c. the best outcome for the greatest number of people possible
d. all of the above
e. two of the above

12. Consistency of image quality may be ascertained through application of
techniques associated with which of the following enabling tools?
1. exposure factors
2. radiographic positioning
3. mAs, kVp, time
4. automatic exposure control
5. film processing
   a. 1, 2
   b. 1, 2, 3
   c. 1, 3, 4
   d. 2, 3, 4, 5
   e. 1, 2, 3, 4, 5

13. Maximizing image quality may be managed through appropriate
processes for outcomes associated with:
a. automatic exposure control
b. total quality improvement (TQI)
c. total quality management (TQM)

    d. a, b

    e. b, c

14. Consistency in radiographic imaging has been greatly enhanced through the application of _____ used with modern equipment.
    a. AEC, APR
    b. a centimeter stick
    c. high-speed screens
    d. communication with the patient
    e. none of the above

15. The most important element of responsibility toward quality patient care is related to:
    a. taking charge of the situation
    b. how we individually respond to others' needs
    c. not responding to what you don't understand
    d. always being on time
    e. accountability for others' work performance

16. Moral responsibility is associated with the concept that individuals are responsible for their own actions.
    a. true
    b. false

17. In the radiology work environment the _____ controls performance related to producing images and the quality of their outcome.
    a. radiologist
    b. radiographer

18. Modern radiology departments are restricted to the use of ionizing radiation producing equipment in the production of radiographic images.
    a. true
    b. false

19. Producing radiographic images is more an art than a science.
    a. true
    b. false

20. Radiographers perform a critical service as a helping profession in the practice of medicine; an element that must be present in the definition of a helping profession is:
    a. modern equipment
    b. human illness, vulnerability
    c. patient communication
    d. professionalism
    e. none of the above

▶ REFERENCES

1. *The American Heritage Dictionary* (2nd college ed.) (1991). Boston: Houghton Mifflin Company.

2. American Society of Radiologic Technologists (1993). *The professional curriculum in radiography*. Albuquerque, NM: Author.

3. Appelbaum, SH (1981). *Stress management for health care professionals*. Rockville, MD: Aspen Publishers.

4. Beabout, GR, & Wennemann, DJ (1994). *Applied professional ethics; A developmental approach for use with case studies*. Lanham, MD: University Press of America, Inc.

5. Fletcher, J (1966). *Situation ethics, the new morality*. Philadelphia: The Westminster Press.

6. Flexner, A (1960). *Medical education in the United States and Canada: A report to the Carnegie Foundation for the advancement of teaching*. Washington, DC: Science and Health Publications, Inc. (Original work published by Carnegie Foundation, New York, 1910.)

7. The Joint Commission on Accreditation of Healthcare Organizations. (1995). *1995 Accreditation manual for hospitals: Vol. 1. Standards*. Oakbrook Terrace, IL: Author.

8. Pellegrino, ED, Thomasma , DC (1993). *The virtues in medical practice*. New York: Oxford University Press.

9. Selye, H (1976). *Stress in health and disease*. Boston: Butterworths.

10. Thomas, CL (Ed.). (1993). *Taber's cyclopedic medical dictionary*. Philadelphia: F. A. Davis.

11. Thompson, MA, Hattaway, MP, Hall, JD, & Dowd, SB (1994). *Principles of imaging science and protection*. Philadelphia: W. B. Saunders.

12. Wolf, SG, Finestone, AG (1986). *Health and performance at work, occupational stress*. Littleton, MA: PSG Publishing Company.

CHAPTER

Professional Role

▶ OBJECTIVES

At the conclusion of the learning opportunity the reader will be able to:

1. Discuss the concept of perception and how it relates to social classes and to the labeling of groups.
2. Discuss professional image and name factors used by groups in equating their discipline to others and comparing two or more disciplines not their own.
3. Define professionalism in Pellegrino's terms.
4. Name the evolutionary stages in the development of a profession according to Borish.
5. Relate cultural image to how professionals present themselves to other professionals and to the public.
6. Discuss where radiologic technologists fit into the health-care environment today.
7. Name the elements of the radiographer's professional role and relate the various elements to statements from radiography's code of ethics.

▶ INTRODUCTION

In the first chapter, elements of the professional role of radiographer were identified. As the book has progressed, the student has been familiarized with what is involved in being a technically competent practitioner, an ethically competent practitioner, a patient-care services provider, an advocate for radiation safety and protection, and a user of initiative and independent judgment in applying radiologic techniques. To broaden the reader's knowledge base, the book has also provided information about the historical background of radiography and also the health-care delivery system, hospitals, and radiology departments.

In this chapter we will first discuss the professional role of radiographer from the perspectives of perception and professional image and then summarize the elements of the professional role. In a sense, it is difficult to separate the concepts of perception and professional image in that perception—both self-perception and the perception of others—is an integral part of a professional image. Professional image will be discussed here in terms of the prevailing self- and public impressions about radiographers, what constitutes professionalism, the evolution of a profession, cultural image, and where radiologic technologists fit in. The intent of this section is to present a multi-sided definition of the professional role of the radiographer in the health-care delivery environment. The last section will define the elements of the professional role in terms of the discipline's code of ethics with the intent that the student will begin to recognize and internalize these elements as criteria for being a "professional" radiographer.

▶ PERCEPTION

"A mental impression of something perceived by the senses together with comprehension of what it is. Perception thus is the act or process of perceiving" [9]. This definition of *perception* conforms with the intent of this chapter. It is important to understand the concepts of perception and professionalism in order to begin to internalize the appropriate image of the radiographer as a professional and understand the various facets of the role.

To illustrate the concept of perception more clearly, let us look at a reference to social structure. In Fussell's [5] book *Class*, a guide to the American status system, the author used a chart to reflect three categories of social class perceived by Americans (Figure 9-1). This chart, although somewhat amusing, clearly illustrates how Americans view each other socially based on material possessions, behavior, and language. Thus, from this frame of reference it seems reasonable to conclude that perception originates in the eye and mind of the beholder.

Further, in *The Unheavenly City, Revisited* Banfield [1] wrote about various aspects of urban crises and, referring to different social classes, said they "share a distinct patterning of attitudes, values and modes of behavior" (p. 56). The writings of Fussell and Banfield reflect similar beliefs about how people are assigned to a social class—that people who live similar lifestyles and who do similar work become collectively labeled (e.g., middle class, proletariat, professionals, working class). Given this method of automatic classification, as groups we become identified largely by the work we do and/or how we are perceived through our behavior. Later we will discuss why some groups are identified as professionals and also why health professionals are set apart from other workers.

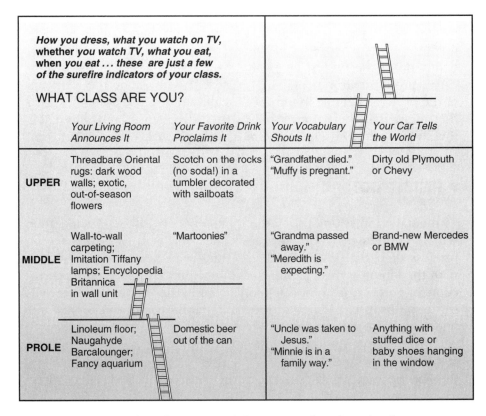

How you dress, what you watch on TV, whether *you watch TV, what you eat,* when *you eat ... these are just a few* of the surefire indicators of your class.

WHAT CLASS ARE YOU?

	Your Living Room Announces It	Your Favorite Drink Proclaims It	Your Vocabulary Shouts It	Your Car Tells the World
UPPER	Threadbare Oriental rugs: dark wood walls; exotic, out-of-season flowers	Scotch on the rocks (no soda!) in a tumbler decorated with sailboats	"Grandfather died." "Muffy is pregnant."	Dirty old Plymouth or Chevy
MIDDLE	Wall-to-wall carpeting; Imitation Tiffany lamps; Encyclopedia Britannica in wall unit	"Martoonies"	"Grandma passed away." "Meredith is expecting."	Brand-new Mercedes or BMW
PROLE	Linoleum floor; Naugahyde Barcalounger; Fancy aquarium	Domestic beer out of the can	"Uncle was taken to Jesus." "Minnie is in a family way."	Anything with stuffed dice or baby shoes hanging in the window

FIGURE 9-1. What class are you? [From Fussel, P (1983). *Class.* New York: Ballantine Books.]

▶ PROFESSIONAL IMAGE

Historically, radiographers have often been perceived as button pushers. This impression may have evolved because persons outside the profession lacked knowledge of the intensity of the educational background prescribed for study of the radiological sciences; radiographers themselves may also have contributed to this impression. Professional image is, in part, projected through both individual behavior and group behavior. How do radiographers themselves perceive their relationship with others in the work environment? How does that perceived relationship affect radiographers' self-esteem? How do radiographers' self-perception and self-esteem influence the way they present themselves to each other, patients, other health-care team members, and the public? In Chapter 2, relationships among practitioners of the various imaging modalities were described as basically those of colleagues or peers; this is a comfortable, nonchallenging relationship in which persons share a common knowledge base and understand what skills are required to perform the duties of specific roles. However, radiographers work in a milieu in which most of their co-workers are also health-care professsionals, many from different disciplines. Do their relationships with practitioners from different disciplines affect how radiographers feel about themselves? The questions posed here represent areas where radiographers need to compare their own image as professionals with that of other health professionals such as nurses. Are radiographers seen as professionals in the same way that nurses are?

In a study reported in the *Radiologic Technology Journal* [7], a group of physical and occupational therapists ranked thirteen allied health professions, including radiologic technologists, in occupational prestige. These allied health professions included audiologists, dental hygienists, dietitians, medical records administrators, medical technologists, occupational therapists, physical therapists, physician assistants, radiologic technologists, rehabilitation counselors, respiratory therapists, social workers, and speech pathologists. The article defined prestige as it relates to the esteem or social status accorded an occupation by the general public. Physical therapists ranked radiologic technologists as thirteenth (score of 58.2) in prestige; occupational therapists ranked them as twelveth (score of 62.1). The physical and occupational therapists generally agreed on their prestige ratings for all thirteen disciplines as reflected in their rankings of radiologic technologists. The authors then compared their findings to the findings from earlier studies conducted by the National Opinion Research Center (NORC) on other occupations. These comparisons, displayed in Table 9-1, clearly show that findings related to the physical therapist and occupational therapist rankings in the Parker and Chan study correlate with findings from the NORC study. The article suggests that a consensus extracted from previous articles infers that such factors as training, education, knowledge required, monetary rewards, and the nature of the work (authority, responsibility and security) (p. 152) are the contributing factors used by groups to equate their discipline to others. It can be postulated that these same factors may be used by groups in equating or comparing two or more disciplines not their own; however, this supposition is merely speculative

TABLE 9-1

Rankings of Radiographers in Prestige by Physical Therapists and Occupational Therapists. Comparison with Previous NORC Studies

Occupation	Prestige Score
Supreme court justice	96 and 94
Public school teacher	78 and 91
Accountant/sociologist	Low 80s
Plumber, auto repairman, barber	Mid 60s
Store clerk/truck driver	High 50s
Rad tech prestige score (from Parker-Chan study)	58.2 and 62.1

at this point. Nevertheless, the results reported in the Parker and Chan study show that radiologic technologists need to be better communicators about how their discipline equates favorably with others in terms of education and knowledge required to be a radiologic technologist as well as the responsibilities and authorities delegated through that professional role.

To look at the factors of perceptions and class from another angle, let us consider a seeming correlation between descriptions appearing in the chapter "The Imperatives of Class" [1] and the past behavior of radiologic technologists. Banfield explains characteristics of class behavior based on the consequences of a time horizon theory; that is, certain classes of people live present-oriented or future-oriented lifestyles. In this context, the time-horizon theory relates to certain traits of a lifestyle or culture and may be best understood as resulting from more or less ability or desire to prepare for the future (p. 56). Application of this theory is not intended to illustrate the complexities of class culture or the individuals therein. If, however, social class culture were placed on a scale of how much people invest in the future, the upper class would be at the high (future-oriented) end and the lower class at the lower (present-oriented) end. Figure 9-2 is a simple portrayal of a social class scale based on incentives (e.g., education) and motivation.

The upper and middle classes differ to some degree in commitment to community and organizations. However, in both groups expectations run very high and both have many opportunities avail-

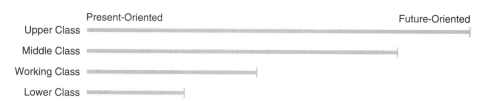

FIGURE 9-2.   Social class scale based on incentives and motivation.

able; thus, they prepare for a secure future for themselves and their children.

The working class does not invest much in the future but measures life by luck, hard work, discipline, and family attachments and assumes that old age is middle age. The present-oriented lower class expects life to offer few opportunities and involuntarily lives moment to moment, with little or no incentive for relief.

There may be various reasons why radiologic technologists have not achieved the occupational prestige level of other health professionals after more than 75 years of involvement in health care. However, it seems clear that the discipline made very few advances in the curriculum for nearly 50 years. Until the early 1970s, when technology began a dynamic growth, there was little for radiologic technologists to look forward to in terms of career advancement and a limited educational basis by which to compare themselves to other disciplines. Even though educational curriculum parameters have existed historically, the curriculum actually taught was seriously abbreviated because of a short-term, job-oriented philosophy. Thus, few radiographers made an investment in advanced education, believing that the education gained in becoming licensed and certified and on the job was sufficient for what they needed to know. This definitely has changed so that the radiological sciences disciplines are advancing to educational levels comparable to any other health-care profession. We only need to change our goals, attitude, behavior, and self-perception accordingly.

Professionalism

Professionalism refers to the conduct, aims, or qualities that characterize or make a profession or a professional person. Pellegrino [8] described true professions as those that deal with humans "(1) when they are most vulnerable, (2) when they lack the knowledge to make their own decisions, and (3) when a relationship is not of equal power, because all the knowledge is on one side and the need for help is on the other side" (p. 172). Many occupations that were once regarded as crafts, arts, trades, and commerce have come to claim many elements associated with traditional true professions. For example, most occupations "set standards for entry, establish educational requirements and curriculum, form national organizations, publish a journal or magazine, set fees and standards of performance, and usually establish codes of ethics" (p. 171). All of these standards, however, are social standards. Those precepts that constitute higher moral and ethical codes come from philosophical definitions created by the special nature of human relations when people are vulnerable and in need. This specialness sets health professionals apart from other professionals.

Development of a Profession

"The clearly marked evolutionary stages of the birth of a profession are the development of specialized skills, the development of a humane and elevated ethical code, and the winning of the ethical respect of society as an honorific vocation" [3, p. 22].

Radiography is a highly specialized discipline with many clinical specialties, administrators, and educators, and the discipline has established a very humane code of ethics. The question remains, however: Does society hold ethical respect for radiographers? Does society know who we are or what we do? If not, who will communicate the message and how will the message be communicated? In seeking answers, let us look at the issue of image from a cultural aspect.

Cultural Image

What we see is what we get. Well, not necessarily. But what we see may determine how we perceive. In *The Professional Image*, Bixler [2, pp. 20–21] describes a mural called "Modifications of Soft Tissue" that hangs in the Smithsonian Institute in Washington, DC. The mural, which depicts a world of cultural practices that reflect the importance and power of image, includes representations of the following historical cultural customs.

1. Chinese women are shown with bound, crippled feet or "golden lilies." This practice marked them as elite and removed from the ordinary manual labor class. They adorned the environment.

2. New Guinea men are presented with scarification on their skin; the scarring was viewed as revealing manhood.

3. In the Congo of Africa, the inhabitants are portrayed with cone-shaped heads, which was achieved by binding infants' heads tightly.

4. Wealthy women of Burma and Thailand are depicted with bands placed around their necks to stretch the muscles so that they atrophied. If the bands were removed, the neck broke (a powerful control for a husband).

The visible signs just described are associated with culturally diverse messages of perceived beauty, prestige, power, or desirability. Visual messages such as body language, personal grooming, and the clothes we wear are also a factor in nonverbal communication. Facial expressions, eye contact, and mannerisms such as fidgeting all send messages related to self-confidence and maturity.

People should be proud of the work they do. If they are not proud, or for some other reason are unhappy with their work, they will not experience the boost in self-esteem that comes from the feeling of being productive and that a job has been well done. If the job itself is not valued, if the person performing it does not see worth in what he or she is doing, it is difficult for that person to respect self, the workplace, or the persons served.

If we feel dissatisfied with what we do and think that our role as radiographers in health-care delivery is not as important as other roles, we are not likely to project self-confidence through the polite, assured attitude of the professional; this type of attitude always reflects an element of warm and caring respect for those in need.

Building self-esteem requires a personal commitment to whatever one is doing. In order to have a commitment in radiography, we have to be able to see ourselves in a global perspective. In a 1964 *Harvard Business Review* article, "The Power to See Ourselves," the author, Paul J. Brouwer [4], explained that a factor in the dynamics of growth is that people must see themselves as part of their whole environment—that they must develop a self-image both personal and impersonal in response to what they see around them. Brouwer's advice is as true today as it was in 1964. It is time that radiographers act on this advice and strive to see themselves from a global perspective.

Individuals must ask if their world is small (as a child's is) or if they relate to the environment, events, and other people in a more global fashion? Everyone has his or her point of view, and radiographers must exhibit a respect for others' thinking as well as the ability to think independently and knowledgeably on their own. Radiographers are intelligent, hard-working professionals who undergo a relatively intense curriculum and deserve a great deal of respect. Historically, radiographers have not collectively commanded that respect because some of their behavior has reflected a lack of understanding of the value of their professional role in health care as well as a lack of personal self-esteem. Radiographers are the only ones who can change how they are perceived and they can do this by focusing on the value of their professional role and concentrating their efforts on being the type of professional who commands respect from colleagues and the public.

Where Do Radiologic Technologists Fit in?

Although allied health professions vary in scope of practice, it is very clear that practitioners of disciplines such as radiologic technology are true professionals because their responsibilities and functions bring them in direct personal contact with persons when they are ill and vulnerable as patients. Radiologic technologists therefore must strive to maintain the high expectations and moral obligations as set forth by the original humane professions of medicine, law, and theology.

As previously stated, a true profession is not determined by legal or social definitions but by the nature of the service provided and the situation of persons who need the service [8]. The fact that people who are ill and/or seeking health care are vulnerable and in need is made manifest in the following quote.

> To be sure, the poor, the imprisoned, the lonely, and the rejected are also deprived of the full expression of their humanity, so much so, that men in these conditions may long for death to liberate them. But none save saints seek illness as a road to liberation. The poor man can

still hope for a change of fortune, the prisoner for a reprieve, the lonely for a friend. But the ill person remains impaired when freed of these other constraints on the free exercise of his humanity. [6, p. 159]

▶ PROFESSIONAL ROLE

Although this book has presented a new terminology and specific definitions for the elements of the professional role of the radiologic technologist, the elements themselves directly relate to the "Code of Ethics for the Profession of Radiologic Technology" (see Chapter 8). More than just a code of ethics, this document establishes standards for the elements we have assigned to the professional role. In the section that follows, the elements are defined in terms of the appropriate statements from the radiography code of ethics (numbers in parentheses are the numbers of the relevant statement).

Technically Competent Practitioner

As a technically competent practitioner, the radiologic technologist "practices technology founded upon theoretical knowledge and concepts, utilizes equipment and accessories consistent with the purpose for which they have been designed, and employs procedures and techniques appropriately" (4); and "continually strives to improve knowledge and skills by participating in educational and professional activities, sharing knowledge with colleagues and investigating new and innovative aspects of professional practice" (10).

Ethically Competent Practitioner

As an ethically competent practitioner, the radiologic technologist "acts to advance the principal objective of the profession to provide services to humanity with full respect for the dignity of mankind" (2); "practices ethical conduct appropriate to the profession, and protects the patient's right to quality radiologic technology care" (8); and "respects confidences entrusted in the course of professional practice, protects the patient's right to privacy, and reveals confidential information only as required by law or to protect the welfare of the individual or the community" (9).

Patient-Care Services Provider

As a patient-care services provider the radiologic technologist "conducts himself/herself in a professional manner, responds to patient needs and supports colleagues and associates in providing quality patient care" (1); "delivers patient care and service unrestricted by concerns of personal attributes or the nature of the disease or illness, and without discrimination, regardless of sex, race, creed, religion or socioeconomic status" (3); and "acts as an agent through observation and communication to obtain pertinent information for the physician to aid in the diagnosis and treatment management of the patient, and recognizes that interpretation and diagnosis are outside the scope of practice for the profession" (6).

Advocate for Radiation Safety and Protection

As an advocate for radiation safety and protection, the radiologic technologist "utilizes equipment and accessories, employs techniques and procedures, performs services in accordance with an accepted standard of practice, and demonstrates expertise in limiting the radiation exposure to the patient, self, and other members of the health-care team" (7).

User of Initiative and Independent Judgment in Applying Radiologic Techniques and Radiation Protection Measures

As a user of initiative and independent judgment in applying radiologic techniques and radiation protection measures, the radiologic technologist "assesses situations; exercises care, discretion, and judgment; assumes responsibility for professional decisions; and acts in the best interest of the patient" (5).

► CONCLUSION

This chapter has presented a wide range of ideas relating to perception, professional image, and professional role and has included discussions on professionalism, development of professions, cultural image, and how the role of radiologic technologist fits into the framework of a profession. Examples cited from the literature represent those the author has found meaningful in her own studies and work/life experiences. A sincere attempt has been made throughout the book to illustrate who radiologic technologists are, where they came from, what they do, how they can control their work environment, what it means to act ethically and professionally, and why they are a vital and essential component of the health-care team in an ever-changing health-care delivery system.

TEST QUESTIONS

1. People may view others socially according to the language they use, their behavior, and/or their possessions.
   a. true
   b. false

2. The studies of Fussell and Banfield suggest that people are assigned to a social class by others through collective labeling (automatic classification).
   a. true
   b. false

3. Professional image is in part projected through:
   1. individual behavior
   2. collective labeling
   3. group behavior
   4. material possessions
      a. 1, 2
      b. 2, 3
      c. 1, 3
      d. 2, 4
      e. 1, 2, 3, and 4

4. Success in the social and work worlds may be largely contingent on such criteria as:
   a. preparation for the future
   b. education
   c. being a member of the upper class
   d. a and b
   e. a, b, and c

5. As defined by Pellegrino, those elements that characterize true professions include:
   a. work that deals with human beings
   b. the vulnerability of sick people
   c. an unequal power of knowledge
   d. a and c only
   e. a, b, and c

6. Standards of performance that constitute higher moral standards are largely based in the precepts of:
   a. social standards
   b. philosophical standards

7. Development of a profession evolves through several stages that are associated with:
   a. perception by the public as honorable work
   b. specialized skills
   c. written humane ethical code
   d. b and c only
   e. all of the above

8. The perceived power of cultural image is reflected in representations determined through important practices associated with:
   a. prestige and power
   b. beauty and desirability
   c. gender and race
   d. a and b only
   e. all of the above

9. It is important for radiologic technologists to view themselves as a part of the global world of health-care delivery professionals.
   a. true
   b. false

10. The primary reason that radiologic techhnologists are associated with the true professions of medicine, law, and theology is because:
    a. they have direct personal contact with persons who are ill
    b. they observe legal and social standards
    c. people who are ill are vulnerable
    d. a only
    e. a, b, and c

11. The elements of the professional role of radiologic technologist relate directly to the Code of Ethics for the Profession of Radiologic Technology.
    a. true
    b. false

Essay Question

12. Write a brief paragraph expressing your understanding of a) what the professional role of the radiographer is, b) what a true professional is, c) why the radiographer is a true professional, d) how perception can affect the way in which the profession is viewed, and e) why the profession is an important component of the health-care delivery team.

▶ REFERENCES

1. Banfield, EC (1974). *The unheavenly city revisited*. Boston: Little Brown and Company.

2. Bixler, S (1984). *The professional image*. New York: Perigee Books. The Putnam Group.

3. Borish, IM (1983). The academy and professionalism. *The American Academy of Optometry, 57*(2), 18-23.

4. Brouwer, P (1964). The power to see ourselves. *Harvard Business Review, 42*(6), 156.

5. Fussell, P (1983). *Class*. New York: Ballantine Books.

6. Kastenbaum, V (Ed). (1982). *The humanity of the ill*. Knoxville: University of Tennessee Press.

7. Parker, HJ, Chan, F (1985). Prestige of radiologic technologists. *Radiologic Technology, 57*(2), 152-156.

8. Pellegrino, ED (1983). What is a profession? *Journal of Allied Health, August*, pp. 168-176.

9. *Webster's II New Riverside Dictionary*. (1984). New York: Berkeley Books.

APPENDIX

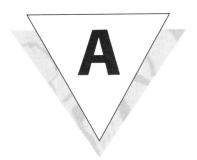

A

Radiography Standards of Practice*

▶ INTRODUCTION

The complex nature of disease processes involves multiple imaging modalities. Although an interdisciplinary team of radiologists, radiographers and support staff plays a critical role in the delivery of health services, it is the radiographer who performs the radiographic examination that creates the images needed for diagnosis. Radiography integrates scientific knowledge and technical skills with effective patient interaction to provide quality patient care and informative diagnostic information.

Radiographer

The radiographer must demonstrate an understanding of human anatomy, physiology, pathology and medical terminology.

---

*Reprinted with permission of the American Society of Radiologic Technologists. All rights reserved. Copyrighted, 1998.

The radiographer must maintain a high degree of accuracy in radiographic positioning and exposure technique. Knowledge must be maintained in the areas of radiation protection and safety. Radiographers prepare for and assist the radiologist in the completion of intricate radiographic examinations. They prepare and administer contrast media and medications in accordance with state and federal regulations.

The radiographer is the primary liaison between patients and radiologists and other members of the support team. They must remain sensitive to the physical and emotional needs of the patient through good communication, patient assessment, patient monitoring and patient care skills.

The radiographer uses professional and ethical judgment and critical thinking when performing their duties. Quality improvement and customer service allows the radiographer to be a responsible member of the health care team by continually assessing professional performance. The radiographer is involved with patient education to provide optimal care, public education regarding the profession and continuing education to enhance their knowledge and technical competence.

Education and Certification

Radiographers prepare for their role on the interdisciplinary team by satisfactorily completing an educational program in radiologic technology. Two-year certificate, associate degree and four-year baccalaureate degree programs exist throughout the United States.

Accredited programs must meet specific curricular and educational standards. The Joint Review Committee on Education in Radiologic Technology (JRCERT) is the accrediting agency for radiologic technology programs recognized by the U.S. Department of Education.

Upon completion of a course of study in radiologic technology, individuals may apply to take the national certification examination. The American Registry of Radiologic Technologists (ARRT) is the recognized certifying agency for radiographers and offers an examination three times per year. Those who successfully complete the certification examination in radiography may use the credential R.T. (R) following their name; the R.T. signifies registered technologist and the (R) indicates radiography. To maintain ARRT certification and a level of expertise and awareness of changes and advances in practice, radiologic technologists must complete 24 hours of appropriate continuing education every two years.

▶ RADIOGRAPHY STANDARDS OF PRACTICE

Standard One–Assessment

The practitioner collects pertinent data about the patient and about the procedure.

Rationale.   Information about the patient's health status is essential in providing appropriate imaging and therapeutic services.

General Criteria.   The practitioner:

1. Uses consistent and appropriate techniques to gather relevant information from the medical record, significant others and health care providers. The collection of information is determined by the patient's needs or condition.
2. Reconfirms patient identification and verifies the procedure requested or prescribed.
3. Verifies the patient's pregnancy status, when appropriate.
4. Determines whether the patient has been appropriately prepared for the procedure.
5. Assesses factors that may contraindicate the procedure, such as medications, insufficient patient preparation or artifacts.

Specific Criteria.   The practitioner:

1. Identifies artifact-producing objects such as dentures, chest leads, jewelry and hearing aids.

Standard Two–Analysis/Determination of Action Plan

The practitioner analyzes the information obtained during the assessment phase and develops an action plan for completing the procedure.

Rationale. Determining the most appropriate action plan enhances patient safety and comfort, optimizes diagnostic and therapeutic quality and improves cost effectiveness.

General Criteria. The practitioner:

1. Selects the most appropriate and cost-effective action plan after reviewing all pertinent data and assessing the patient's abilities and condition.
2. Uses his or her professional judgment to adapt imaging and therapeutic procedures to improve diagnostic quality and therapeutic outcome.
3. When necessary, consults appropriate medical personnel to determine a modified action plan.
4. Determines the need for accessory equipment. Determination of the most appropriate action plan optimizes patient safety, comfort, diagnostic and therapeutic quality and cost effectiveness.

Specific Criteria. The practitioner:

1. Evaluates lab values prior to administering contrast media and beginning interventional procedures.
2. Selects appropriate shielding devices.
3. Selects appropriate patient immobilization devices.
4. Determines appropriate type and dose of contrast agent to be administered, based on the patient's age, weight and medical/physical status.
5. Reviews the patient's chart and the physician's request to determine optimal imaging procedure for suspected pathology.

Standard Three—Patient Education

The practitioner provides information about the procedure to the patient, significant others and health care providers.

Rationale. Communication and education are necessary to establish a positive relationship with the patient, significant others and health care providers.

General Critiera.   The practitioner:

1. Verifies that the patient has consented to the procedure and fully understands its risks, benefits, alternatives and follow-up. When appropriate, the practitioner verifies that written consent has been obtained.
2. Provides accurate explanations and instructions at an appropriate time and at a level the patient can understand. Addresses and documents patient questions and concerns regarding the procedure, when appropriate.
3. Refers questions about diagnosis, treatment or prognosis to the patient's physician.
4. Provides appropriate information to any individual involved in the patient's care.

Specific Criteria.   The practitioner:

1. Consults with other departments, such as patient transportation and anesthesia, for patient services.
2. Instructs patients regarding preparation prior to imaging procedures, including providing information about oral or bowel preparation and allergy preparation.
3. Ensures that all procedural requirements are in place to achieve a quality diagnostic examination.
4. Explains precautions regarding administration of contrast agents to nursing mothers.

Standard Four—Implementation of Action Plan

The practitioner implements the action plan.

Rationale.   Quality patient services are provided through the safe and accurate implementation of a deliberate plan of action.

General Criteria.   The practitioner:

1. Implements an action plan that falls within established protocols and guidelines.
2. Elicits the cooperation of the patient to carry out the action plan.

3. Uses an integrated team approach as needed.
4. Modifies the action plan according to changes in clinical situation.
5. Administers first aid or provides life support in emergency situations.
6. Uses accessory equipment when appropriate.
7. Assesses and monitors the patient's physical and mental status.

Specific Criteria.   The practitioner:

1. Performs venipuncture, IV patency and maintenance procedures according to established guidelines.
2. Administers contrast agents according to established guidelines.
3. Monitors the patient for reactions to contrast agent.
4. Uses appropriate radiation safety devices.
5. Monitors the patient's physical condition during the procedure.
6. Applies appropriate patient immobilization devices when necessary.

Standard Five—Evaluation

The practitioner determines whether the goals of the action plan have been achieved.

Rationale.   Careful examination of the procedure is necessary to determine that all goals have been met.

General Criteria.   The practitioner:

1. Evaluates the patient and the procedure to identify variances that may affect patient outcome. The evaluation process should be timely, accurate and comprehensive.
2. Measures the procedure against established protocols and guidelines.
3. Identifies any exceptions to the expected outcome.

4. Documents any exceptions clearly and completely.
5. If necessary, develops a revised action plan to achieve the intended outcome.

Specific Criteria.   The practitioner:

1. Reviews images to determine if additional images will enhance the diagnostic value of the procedure.

Standard Six–Implementation of Revised Action Plan

The practitioner implements the revised action plan.

Rationale.   It may be necessary to make changes to the action plan to achieve the intended outcome.

General Criteria.   The practitioner:

1. Bases the revised action plan on the patient's condition and the most appropriate means of achieving the intended outcome.
2. Takes action based on patient and procedural variances.
3. Measures and evaluates the results of the revised action plan.
4. Notifies appropriate health provider when immediate clinical response is necessary based on procedural findings and patient condition.

Specific Criteria.   None added.

Standard Seven–Outcome Measurement

The practitioner reviews and evaluates the outcome of the procedure.

Rationale.   To evaluate the quality of care, it is necessary to compare the actual outcome with the intended outcome.

General Criteria.   The practitioner:

1. Reviews all diagnostic/therapeutic data for completeness and accuracy.
2. Determines whether the actual outcome is within the established criteria.
3. Evaluates the process and recognizes opportunities for future changes.
4. Assesses the patient's physical and mental status prior to discharge from the practitioner's care.

Specific Criteria. None added.

Standard Eight–Documentation

The practitioner documents information about patient care, the procedure and the final outcome.

Rationale. Clear and precise documentation is essential for continuity of care, accuracy of care and quality assurance.

General Criteria. The practitioner:

1. Documents diagnostic, treatment and patient data in the appropriate record. Documentation must be timely, accurate, concise and complete.
2. Documents any exceptions from the established criteria or procedures.
3. Records diagnostic or treatment data.

Specific Criteria. None added.

▶ QUALITY PERFORMANCE STANDARDS

Standard One–Assessment

The practitioner collects pertinent information regarding equipment, the procedure and the work environment.

Rationale. The planning and provision of safe and effective medical services relies on the collection of pertinent information about equipment, procedures and the work environment.

General Criteria. The practitioner:

1. Ensures that services are performed in a safe environment in accordance with established guidelines.
2. Ensures that equipment maintenance and operation comply with established guidelines.
3. Assesses equipment to determine acceptable performance based on established guidelines.
4. Ensures that protocol and procedure manuals include recommended criteria and are reviewed and revised on a regular basis.

Specific Criteria. The practitioner:

1. Maintains controlled access to restricted area during radiation exposure to ensure safety of patients, visitors and hospital personnel.

Standard Two—Analysis/Determination

The practitioner analyzes information collected during the assessment phase and determines whether changes need to be made to equipment, procedures or the work environment.

Rationale. Determination of acceptable performance is necessary for the provision of safe and effective services.

General Criteria. The practitioner:

1. Assesses whether services, procedures and the work environment meet or exceed established guidelines. If not, the practitioner must develop an action plan.
2. Evaluates equipment to determine if it meets or exceeds established standards. If not, the practitioner must develop an action plan.

3. Analyzes information collected during the assessment phase to determine whether optimal services are being provided. If not, the practitioner must develop an action plan.

Specific Criteria. None added.

Standard Three—Education

The practitioner informs patients, the public and other health care providers about procedures, equipment and facilities.

Rationale. Open communication promotes safe practices.

General Criteria. The practitioner:

1. Elicits confidence and cooperation from the patient, the public and health care providers by providing timely communication and effective instruction.
2. Presents explanations and instructions at the learner's level of understanding and learning style.

Specific Criteria. The practitioner:

1. Instructs health care providers or students regarding radiographic procedures and radiation safety.
2. Educates the public about radiographic procedures and radiation safety.

Standard Four—Performance

The practitioner performs quality assurance activities or acquires information on equipment and materials.

Rationale. Quality assurance activities provide valid and reliable information regarding the performance of materials and equipment.

General Criteria. The practitioner:

1. Performs quality assurance activities based on established protocols.
2. Provides evidence of ongoing quality assurance activities.

Specific Criteria.   The practitioner:

1. Monitors image production to determine variance from established quality standards.

Standard Five—Evaluation

The practitioner evaluates quality assurance results and establishes an appropriate action plan.

Rationale.   Materials, equipment and procedure safety depend upon ongoing quality assurance activities that evaluate performance based on established guidelines.

General Criteria.   The practitioner:

1. Compares quality assurance results to established acceptable values.
2. Verifies quality assurance testing conditions and results.
3. Formulates an action plan following verification of testing.

Specific Criteria.   None added.

Standard Six—Implementation

The practitioner implements the quality assurance action plan.

Rationale.   Implementation of a quality assurance action plan is imperative for quality diagnostic and therapeutic procedures and patient care.

General Criteria.   The practitioner:

1. Obtains assistance from appropriate personnel to implement the quality assurance action plan.
2. Implements the quality assurance action plan.

Specific Criteria.   None added.

Standard Seven—Outcome Measurement

The practitioner assesses the outcome of the quality assurance action plan in accordance with established guidelines.

Rationale.   Outcome assessment is an integral part of the on-going quality assurance plan to enhance diagnostic and therapeutic services.

General Criteria.   The practitioner:

1. Reviews the implementation process for accuracy and validity.
2. Based on outcome assessment, determines whether the performance level of equipment and materials is safe for practice.
3. Develops and implements a modified action plan when testing results are not in compliance with guidelines.

Specific Criteria.   None added.

Standard Eight—Documentation

The practitioner documents quality assurance activities and results.

Rationale.   Documentation provides evidence of quality assurance activities designed to enhance the safety of patients, the public and health care providers during diagnostic and therapeutic services.

General Criteria.   The practitioner:

1. Maintains documentation of quality assurance activities, procedures and results in accordance with established guidelines.
2. Provides timely, concise, accurate and complete documentation.
3. Provides documentation which includes current protocol, policy and procedures.

Specific Criteria.   None added.

▶ PROFESSIONAL PERFORMANCE STANDARDS

Standard One–Quality

The practitioner strives to provide optimal care to all patients.

Rationale.   All patients expect and deserve optimal care during diagnosis and treatment.

General Criteria.   The practitioner:

1. Works with others to elevate the quality of care.
2. Participates in quality assurance programs.
3. Adheres to the accepted standards, policies and procedures adopted by the profession and regulated by law.
4. Provides the best possible diagnostic study or therapeutic treatment for each patient by applying professional judgment and discretion.
5. Anticipates and responds to the needs of the patient.

Specific Criteria.   None added.

Standard Two–Self-Assessment

The practitioner evaluates personal performance, knowledge and skills.

Rationale.   Self-assessment is an important tool in professional growth and development.

General Criteria.   The practitioner:

1. Monitors personal work ethics, behaviors and attitudes.
2. Evaluates performance and recognizes opportunities for improvement.
3. Recognizes his or her strengths and uses them to benefit patients, coworkers and the profession.

4. Performs procedures only after receiving appropriate education and training.
5. Recognizes and takes advantage of opportunities for educational growth and improvement in technical and problem-solving skills.
6. Actively participates in professional societies and organizations.

Specific Criteria. None added.

Standard Three—Education

The practitioner acquires and maintains current knowledge in clinical practice.

Rationale. Advancements in medical science require enhancement of knowledge and skills through education.

General Criteria. The practitioner:

1. Has completed the appropriate education related to clinical practice.
2. Maintains appropriate credentials and certification related to clinical practice.
3. Participates in educational activities to enhance knowledge, skills and performance.
4. Shares knowledge and expertise with others.

Specific Criteria. None added.

Standard Four—Collaboration and Collegiality

The practitioner promotes a positive, collaborative practice atmosphere with other members of the health care team.

Rationale. To provide quality patient care, all members of the health care team must communicate effectively and work together efficiently.

General Criteria.   The practitioner:

1. Shares knowledge and expertise with colleagues, peers, students and all members of the health care team.
2. Develops collaborative partnerships with other health care providers in the interest of diagnostic and therapeutic quality and cost effectiveness.

Specific Criteria.   None added.

Standard Five—Ethics

The practitioner adheres to the profession's accepted ethical standards.

Rationale.   All decisions and actions made on behalf of the patient must be based on a sound ethical foundation.

General Criteria.   The practitioner:

1. Provides health care services with respect for the patient's dignity and needs.
2. Acts as a patient advocate to support patients' rights.
3. Takes responsibility for professional decisions.
4. Delivers patient care and service without bias based on personal attributes, nature of the disease, sex, race, creed, religion or socioeconomic status.
5. Respects the patient's right to privacy and confidentiality.
6. Adheres to the established standards of practice of the profession.

Specific Criteria.   None added.

Standard Six—Exploration and Investigation

The practitioner participates in activities that lead to the acquisition, dissemination and advancement of the professional knowledge base.

Rationale.   Scholarly activities such as research, scientific investigation, presentation and publication advance the profession and thereby improve the quality and efficiency of patient services.

General Criteria.   The practitioner:

1. Reads and critically evaluates research in diagnostic and therapeutic services.
2. Investigates new, innovative methods and applies them in practice.
3. Shares information with colleagues through publication, presentation and collaboration.
4. Pursues lifelong learning.
5. Participates in data collection.

Specific Criteria.   None added.

▶ RADIOGRAPHY GLOSSARY

Artifact   False features in the image produced by patient instability or equipment deficiencies.

Assessment   The act of estimating or determining the significance, importance or value of.

Clinical   Pertaining to or found on actual observation and treatment of patients.

Competency   Having the ability to perform a task.

Contrast media   Substance administered to subject being imaged to alter selectively the image intensity of a particular anatomical or functional region.

Contraindicate   To make (the indicated or expected treatment or drug) inadvisable.

Disease   A disorder or abnormal condition having a characteristic train of symptoms that may affect the whole body or any of its parts. Its etiology, pathology and prognosis may be known or unknown.

Ethical   Conforming to the standards of conduct of a given profession or group.

Interpret   To understand and explain an image for purposes of providing a diagnostic report.

Interventional procedures   Percutaneous catheterization for therapeutic purposes.

Quality assurance   A comprehensive set of policies and procedures designed to optimize the performance of personnel and equipment.

Radiation protection   Procedures followed to prevent inappropriate or accidental irradiation of patient, public and health care professionals.

Radiograph   An image produced on a sensitized film by x-rays.

Venipuncture   The puncture of a vein.

APPENDIX

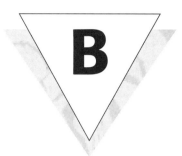

The American Registry of Radiologic Technologists Continuing Education Requirements for Renewal of Registration (January 1997)

SECTION 1. INTRODUCTION

The Board of Trustees of The American Registry of Radiologic Technologists (ARRT) announced in 1991 that it would begin phasing in continuing education requirements for renewal of registration of certificates. This document describes the CE requirements.

Although the requirements are subject to change as the need arises, the major components as described within this document are not expected to change. Terminology used in the text is defined in Section 19 of this document.

SECTION 2. RATIONALE FOR CONTINUING EDUCATION

Certification is a method of assuring the medical community and the public that an individual is qualified by knowledge and skills to practice within the profession. After initial certification, advancing technology and changing job responsibilities may require a technologist to update their knowledge and skills consistent with any new developments in Radiologic Technology.

Continuing education (CE) provides a mechanism for technologists to fulfill their responsibility to maintain competence and prevent professional obsolescence. Participation in continuing education demonstrates accountability to peers, physicians, health care facilities and the public. It also reinforces the Code of Ethics jointly endorsed by The American Registry of Radiologic Technologists and The American Society of Radiologic Technologists (ASRT).

SECTION 3. RENEWAL OF REGISTRATION OF CERTIFICATE

When an ARRT certificate is first issued, it is automatically registered through January 31 of the year immediately succeeding that in which it was awarded. Thereafter, the certificate holder must complete the application for renewal of registration of the certificate on an annual basis. The renewal period is tied to the technologist's birthmonth.

The month prior to a technologist's birthmonth, an application for renewal of registration is mailed by the ARRT. The technologist has until the end of the birthmonth to return the completed application. Prior to the implementation of the mandatory phase of the CE requirements, the renewal process consisted of completion of the renewal application on which the applicant supplies current information and agrees to continue to practice according to the Standards of Ethics. After the implementation of the mandatory CE requirements, the annual renewal of registration will continue. In addition, every other year, the technologist must document participation in CE by listing on the renewal form the CE activities that were completed during the past two year period (i.e., biennium).

SECTION 4. OPTIONS FOR SATISFYING CE REQUIREMENTS DURING A BIENNIUM

There are three options for meeting the CE requirements. Only one option must be met to satisfy the requirements. The options are: (1) earn 24 CE credits which meet the criteria set forth by the ARRT; or

(2) pass an entry-level examination in a discipline not previously passed and for which the individual is eligible; or (3) pass one of the advanced-level examinations not previously passed and for which the individual is eligible. Each of these options is described in further detail in this document.

SECTION 5. BIENNIAL SCHEDULE OF COMPLIANCE

The CE requirements are linked to a biennial (i.e., two year) schedule with the biennium defined in relation to a registrant's birthmonth. The continuing education credits must be earned or the examination option fulfilled within the two years prior to the birthmonth. **There will be a one-time triennium for registrants having an odd numbered birth year. This three year period (triennium) is described in Section 6.** The renewal of registration will continue on an annual basis, with the CE requirements being checked every other year. The two year CE cycle was selected to allow flexibility in fulfilling the requirements (i.e., if no CE could be earned one year, another year was still available). The completion of one biennium will mark the beginning of the next biennium. **Credits earned in one biennium cannot be carried forward into the next biennium.**

SECTION 6. SCHEDULE OF IMPLEMENTATION (BIENNIUM / TRIENNIUM)
(Registrants first certified in 1994 or later refer to Section 7)

The first phase of the implementation schedule began in 1993 with CE reporting on a voluntary basis in 1995. Recognition for compliance with the requirements during the voluntary phase was awarded at the time of renewal in 1995.

The ARRT implemented mandatory CE beginning on the person's birthmonth in 1995. During this initial phase of mandatory CE requirements, CE reporting was staggered so that all registered technologists are not reporting during the same year (i.e., 1997). All technologists certified prior to 1993 who were born in an even-numbered year began a two-year period (biennium) on the first day of their birthmonth in 1995. This biennium will end on the last day of the month preceding the technologist's birthmonth in 1997. All technologists who were born in an odd-numbered year began a three-year period (triennium) on the first day of their birthmonth in 1995. This triennium will end on the last day of the month preceding the technologist's birthmonth in 1998, during which 36 credits of CE activities must be completed. **Modification of the usual two year cycle (biennium), resulting in a three year cycle (triennium), will occur one time only, between 1995 and 1998.** Note that in both cases, biennium and triennium, credits average 12 per year but are not restricted to 12 per year. Satisfying the CE requirements for renewal of registration during the initial implementation of the mandatory phase will require:

BIENNIUM : Even-Numbered Birth year

1. Completion of twenty-four (24) continuing education credits. Twelve (12) credits must be Category A activities. The remaining twelve (12) credits may be either Category A or Category B activities; **or by**
2. Passing an entry-level examination in a discipline not previously passed and for which the individual is eligible [i.e., an ARRT Examination in Radiography, Nuclear Medicine, or Radiation Therapy; the Nuclear Medicine Examination through the Nu-

clear Medicine Technology Certification Board (NMTCB); the Dosimetry Examination through the Medical Dosimetry Certification Board (MDCB); or a certification examination through the American Registry of Diagnostic Medical Sonographers (ARDMS)]; **or by**
3. Passing an ARRT advanced-level examination not previously passed and for which the individual is eligible [i.e., examinations in Mammography, Cardiovascular-Interventional Technology, Magnetic Resonance Imaging, Computed Tomography, or Quality Management].

Example for an Even-Numbered Birth year

Example 6.1: Because a birth date of February 4, 1958, ends with an even-numbered year, a biennium will be assigned beginning on February 1, 1995, and continuing through January 31, 1997. To comply with the mandatory CE requirements, 24 credits of CE must be reported in February of 1997.

TRIENNIUM : Odd-Numbered Birth year

1. Completion of thirty-six (36) continuing education credits. Eighteen (18) credits must be Category A activities. The remaining eighteen (18) credits may be either Category A or Category B activities; **or by**
2. Completion of twelve (12) Category A or B continuing education credits, **PLUS**, passing an entry-level examination in a discipline not previously passed and for which the individual is eligible [i.e., an ARRT Examination in Radiography, Nuclear Medicine, or Radiation Therapy; the Nuclear Medicine Examination through the Nuclear Medicine Technology Certification Board; the Dosimetry Examination through the Medical Dosimetry Certification Board; or a certification examination through the American Registry of Diagnostic Medical Sonographers]; **or by**

3. Completion of twelve (12) Category A or B continuing education credits, **PLUS**, passing an ARRT advanced-level examination not previously passed and for which the individual is eligible [i.e., examinations in Mammography, Cardiovascular-Interventional Technology, Magnetic Resonance Imaging, Computed Tomography, or Quality Management].

Example for an Odd-Numbered Birth year

Example 6.2: Because a birth date of September 24, 1963, ends with an odd-numbered year, a triennium will be assigned beginning on September 1, 1995, and continuing through August 31, 1998. To comply with the mandatory CE requirements, 36 credits of CE must be reported in September of 1998.

Subsequent sections of this document will refer only to the two year period (biennium) since this will be the normal cycle following initial implementation of the mandatory phase.

SECTION 7. CE REQUIREMENTS FOR NEWLY CERTIFIED REGISTRANTS

New registrants will begin the mandatory CE requirements on the first day of their birthmonth in the second year after passing the examination.

Examples for New Registrants

Example 7.1: New Registrants who pass an initial certification examination in 1995 will begin the first biennium on the first day of their birthmonth in 1997.
Example 7.2: New Registrants who pass an initial certification examination in 1996 will begin the first biennium on the first day of their birthmonth in 1998.

Registrants who become registered in additional modalities will maintain the CE schedule established with their initial registration.

SECTION 8. SATISFACTION OF CONTINUING EDUCATION REQUIREMENTS FOR RENEWAL BY EARNING CE CREDITS

One option for satisfying the CE requirements is to earn twenty-four (24) credits of continuing education during the biennium. At least twelve (12) of these credits must be from Category A activities. The other twelve (12) may be from Category A or Category B activities.

The distinction between Category A and Category B activities is not based on the nature of the activity itself, but rather is based upon whether the activity has been reviewed and approved by a Recognized Continuing Education Evaluation Mechanism (RCEEM). A RCEEM is a quality control mechanism for CE activities. **ARRT approved RCEEMs are identified in Section 19.**

The continuing education requirement is not dependent on the number of ARRT certificates held by an individual. For example, a technologist certified in both radiography and radiation therapy technology need earn only 24 credits per biennium.

SECTION 9. SATISFACTION OF CONTINUING EDUCATION REQUIREMENTS FOR RENEWAL BY PASSING AN EXAMINATION

Within a biennium, technologists who pass an entry-level examination for a discipline in which they are not certified and for which they are eligible, or one of the advanced-level examinations that they have not previously passed and for which they are eligible, have met the continuing education requirement for that biennium.

Examples of entry-level examinations that have been approved by the ARRT are:

(1) Radiography through ARRT.

(2) Nuclear Medicine Technology through ARRT or NMTCB.

(3) Radiation Therapy Technology through ARRT.

(4) Dosimetry through MDCB.

(5) Diagnostic Medical Sonography, Vascular Technology, or Diagnostic Cardiac Sonography through the ARDMS.

Examples of approved advanced level examinations are:

(1) Cardiovascular-Interventional Technology through the ARRT.

(2) Mammography through ARRT.

(3) Computed Tomography through ARRT.

(4) Magnetic Resonance Imaging through ARRT.

(5) Quality Management through ARRT.

SECTION 10. FAILURE TO RENEW REGISTRATION OF A CERTIFICATE

Currently, a technologist who fails to apply for renewal of registration or who does not pay the annual fee is considered no longer registered by the ARRT. Present or prospective employers or state licensing agencies inquiring about the status of such a person will be told that the individual is not registered by the ARRT. Since information for those who do not annually register can quickly become outdated and since providing such information is a service reserved only for registrants, no information on the person (other than that they are not registered by the ARRT) will be provided by the ARRT. *(See Section 12 for information on reinstatement requirements.)*

SECTION 11. PROBATION STATUS: APPLICANTS FOR RENEWAL WHO FAIL TO MEET THE MANDATORY CE REQUIREMENTS

Beginning in 1997, a technologist who applies for renewal of registration of a certificate, but who fails to meet the CE requirements within the previous biennium, will automatically be transferred to a "CE probation" status. Individuals who are on probation due to failure to meet the CE requirements will receive a credential indicating CE probation. This status will be reported in response to any inquiries regarding the technologist's standing with the ARRT.

Technologists who have annually registered but are classified as being on probation due to not meeting the CE requirements may be removed from probation status by successfully completing one of the following options <u>during the first 12 months of the following biennium</u>: an entry-level examination in a different discipline for which they are eligible; or an ARRT advanced-level examination for which they are eligible; or continuing education credits. If the continuing education option is used, the registrant will be required to complete 12 CE credits plus the number of credits lacking from the 24 credits required during the previous biennium, up to a maximum of 24 credits.

Examples of the Number of CE Credits Required for Removal from CE Probation Status (if assigned a biennium)

Example 11.1:	
CE Credits Lacking	*Probation Credits*
2	$12+2 = 14$
6	$12+6 = 18$
9	$12+9 = 21$
12 or more	$12+12 = 24$

Examples of the Number of CE Credits Required for Removal from CE Probation Status (if assigned a triennium)

Example 11.2:

CE Credits Lacking	Probation Credits
2	$12+2 = 14$
10	$12+10 = 22$
18	$12+18 = 30$
24 or more	$12+24 = 36$

In addition to the continuing education credits that are required during the first 12 months of the next biennium for removal from probation status, an additional 24 CE credits must be completed by the end of the biennium in order to remain in compliance with the requirements.

Example of Probation Status

Example 11.3:

June 1, 1997-Registrant with a June birthmonth completed 19 CE credits of the 24 required for the past biennium (lacking 5 credits) and paid the annual registration fee. Placed on probation status.

May 31, 1998-Completed a total of 17 probation CE credits (number lacking [i.e., 5] plus 12) or passed an exam between June 1, 1997, and May 31, 1998, and paid the annual renewal fee.   Removed from probation status.

May 31, 1999-During the 1997-1999 biennium (in addition to the probationary CE requirements) must have completed an additional 24 credits of CE or passed an additional exam and paid the annual fee to remain registered.

A certificate on CE probation that has not been brought into complete compliance to the satisfaction of the ARRT within one (1) year, will be considered as no longer registered by the ARRT.

SECTION 12. REINSTATEMENT OF REGISTRATION OF A CERTIFICATE

All ARRT certified technologists have been assigned a CE biennium

or triennium cycle.   Determining what continuing education will be required if a technologists requests reinstatement will be based upon these assigned dates. (*SEE Section 6 of this document.*)

CE will be required as follows:

(1)   Reinstatement requested prior to the biennium/triennium ending date.
Reinstatement will be allowed without reporting CE if the technologist meets all other eligibility requirements for registration.   CE credits must be reported with the Application for Renewal at the end of the biennium/triennium.

(2)   Reinstatement requested within one year after the biennium/triennium ending date.
    (a)   Report 24 CE credits [or 36 if assigned a triennium] completed during the previous biennium/triennium that was assigned.
        OR
    (b)   Apply for reinstatement under the CE probation status.   CE credits completed during the previous biennium/triennium   may be reported. *(See Section 11 for information on removal from CE probation)*

(3)   Reinstatement requested more than one year after the biennium/triennium ending date.
Reinstatement will not be allowed without successful re-examination in a base discipline in which the technologist is eligible (radiography, nuclear medicine, or radiation therapy technology).

SECTION 13. RETIRED STATUS

The CE requirements apply to ARRT registered technologists who are actively practicing in the profession and to technologists who are not currently practicing, but who either plan to return to active practice or who think that return to active practice is a possibility. Registrants who are permanently retired from the profession

of radiologic technology may apply for retired status. Eligibility for retired status requires that the technologist sign an agreement not to engage to any extent whatsoever in actual patient contact in the provision of medical imaging or radiation therapy, in management of medical imaging or radiation therapy services, in education of persons involved or seeking to become involved in medical imaging or radiation therapy, in commercial sales, services or applications with respect to any aspect of medical imaging or radiation therapy or items, services, or devices used in that technology.   Registrants awarded the retired status may designate themselves as "R.T. (Retired)(ARRT)" and are exempt from the CE requirements.   To maintain registration under the retired status, the annual Application for Renewal and fees must be submitted.   To return to nonretired, registered status, a technologist would be required to comply with the reinstatement procedures outlined in Section 12.

SECTION 14. REQUIREMENTS FOR CONTINUING EDUCATION ACTIVITIES

All activities applied toward the CE requirements must meet the ARRT's definition of a continuing education activity.   The definition states that a learning activity must be planned, organized and administered to enhance the knowledge and skills underlying the professional performance that a technologist uses to provide services to patients, the public, or the medical profession. Activities meeting this definition may be either Category A or Category B depending upon whether they have been approved by a RCEEM. The RCEEM acts as a quality control mechanism for the CE activities.

The individual participating in the CE activity typically does not submit the activity to a RCEEM for approval.   The individual selects activities that have already been submitted to a RCEEM by the sponsor of the activity and have subsequently been approved by the RCEEM.

There are a number of activities that do not require submission to a RCEEM to qualify for Category A credit. They include:

(1.) Activities meeting ARRT's definition of an Approved Academic Course;

(2.) CPR certification through the Heart Association or Red Cross; and

(3.) Activities that have been approved by the American Medical Association (AMA Category 1) or the American Nurses Association (ANA) through the American Nurses Credentialing Center (ANCC), as long as they are relevant to the radiologic sciences.

All other CE activities must be approved by a RCEEM in order to be assigned Category A credits. The ARRT does recognize that some states have legislation requiring CE credits to maintain a state license to practice in the profession. An ARRT registrant who completes CE activities in the state in which he or she is licensed as part of his or her state's licensing requirements may count the CE credit as Category A if the state regulatory agency is mandated by law to evaluate CE activities for licensing purposes. The state licensing agencies currently approved as meeting ARRT criteria are: Florida, Illinois, Iowa, Kentucky, Massachusetts, New Mexico, and Oregon.

Activities that an individual intends to use for Category B credits must satisfy the ARRT's definition as a continuing education activity even though they have not been submitted to a RCEEM for approval. In other words, even though the activity does not involve the peer review procedures provided by a RCEEM, the activity

must be a legitimate continuing education activity (See Section 19, Continuing Education Activity).

SECTION 15. AWARDING OF CREDITS

Category A activities as identified in Section 14 are awarded the number of CE credits assigned by the evaluation mechanism (i.e., RCEEM, state organization) or as specified in this section. Activities not submitted to a RCEEM for approval but which meet the ARRT's definition of a CE activity, will be awarded one (1) CE credit for each contact hour. A contact hour is defined as being equal to 50 to 60 minutes. Activities longer than one hour should be assigned whole or partial CE credit based on the 60 minute hour. Educational activities of 30 to 49 minutes in duration will be awarded one-half CE credit. Activities lasting less than 30 minutes will receive no credit.

Activities meeting the definition of an Approved Academic Course will be awarded credit at the rate of 12 CE credits for each academic quarter credit and 16 CE credits for each academic semester credit. An official transcript indicating a grade of "C" or better is required to receive CE credit for an academic course.

Basic CPR certification will be awarded 3 CE credits with a valid CPR card, limited to 3 credits per biennium. Advanced Life Support, Instructor, or Instructor Trainer CPR certification will be awarded 6 CE credits with a valid advanced CPR card. The total number of credits from CPR certification is limited to 6 CE credits per biennium.

SECTION 16. DOCUMENTATION OF PARTICIPATION IN CE

A Registrant is required to maintain proof of participation in continuing education activities. At

the end of a biennium or reporting period, the ARRT will provide a CE Report Form along with the Application for Renewal of Registration. The registrant will be required to list the completed CE activities on the CE Report Form and attest to the truthfulness of the information. Individual CE documentation forms verifying participation should NOT be returned with the renewal form.

When the CE Report Form is received in the ARRT office, a random sample of registrants will be selected and asked to provide copies of documentation of CE participation. This documentation will be used to verify the CE activities that were reported. Failure to provide documentation acceptable to the ARRT will result in CE probation status. (See Section 11 for additional information on CE probation status.) The ARRT reserves the right to request original documentation when in its sole opinion there is any question regarding authenticity. If original documentation is requested, it will be returned at the end of the inquiry. Original documents should be kept by the technologist for one full year after the end of the biennium or triennium.

A Registrant may decide to have documentation of participation in CE maintained by an ARRT approved record keeping mechanism. Several such mechanisms exist and are provided by various national societies either as a service to members or at a fee to non-members. The ARRT currently recognizes the CE record provided by the ASRT, the SNM-TS, and the state licensing agencies in Florida, Illinois, Iowa, and Kentucky. IT REMAINS THE RESPONSIBILITY OF THE INDIVIDUAL TECHNOLOGIST TO SEE THAT RECORDS ARE MAINTAINED PROPERLY. Errors made by a record keeping mechanism are not acceptable reasons for failure to provide appropriate documentation.

Documentation of participation in Category A continuing education activities must be on a form that clearly indicates the information needed to identify the activity as having been approved by a RCEEM. Documentation must include name of the participant, dates of attendance, title and content of the activity, number of contact hours for the activity, name of the sponsor, signature of the instructor or an authorized representative of the sponsor issuing the documentation, and CE reference number. A copy of a college transcript serves as sufficient documentation for Approved Academic Courses as defined by the ARRT. A valid certification card in Basic Life Support, Advanced Life Support, Instructor, or Instructor Trainer from the Red Cross or the American Heart Association is required to receive credit for continuing education in CPR (See Section 19 for definitions of an Approved Academic Course and CPR).

Documentation of participation in Category B activities must be on an itemized form and must include name of participant, dates of attendance, title and content of the activity, number of contact hours for the activity, name of sponsor, and the signature of the instructor or an authorized representative of the sponsor issuing the documentation.

SECTION 17. REQUIREMENTS FOR CE SPONSORS

Sponsors of continuing education activities are responsible for the content, quality and integrity of the educational activity. Sponsors plan, organize, support, endorse, subsidize and/or administer educational activities. Sponsors are also responsible to document participation by the attendees for possible verification at a later date. Sponsors may be, but are not limited to, national, regional, state, and district professional societies, academic institutions, health care agencies, health care facilities, federal, state, and local government agencies or individuals. Sponsors must apply for and receive approval from a RCEEM in order to award Category A credit for activities. Other activities offered by a sponsor that meet the ARRT's definition of continuing education may be assigned Category B credit.

SECTION 18. RESPONSIBILITY OF THE REGISTERED TECHNOLOGIST

COMPLIANCE WITH THE CE REQUIREMENTS IS ULTIMATELY THE INDIVIDUAL'S RESPONSIBILITY. If an activity is intended for use as Category A credit, the technologist is responsible for contacting the sponsor of the CE activity if there are questions as to whether the activity has been approved by a RCEEM. If the examination option is going to be attempted, the technologist must make sure that sufficient time is available to comply with the CE requirements in the event that the examination is not passed.

THE TECHNOLOGIST IS RESPONSIBLE FOR MAINTAINING PROPER DOCUMENTATION ON ACTIVITIES EVEN IF AN ARRT APPROVED RECORD KEEPING MECHANISM IS BEING UTILIZED TO TRACK CREDITS. As noted in Section 16, the technologist is also responsible for providing proper documentation at the request of the ARRT for validation of CE participation.

SECTION 19. DEFINITION OF TERMS

Terminology used within this document is defined as follows:

ACR: American College of Radiology

AHRA: American Healthcare Radiology Administrators

Approved Academic Course: A formal course of study that is relevant to the radiologic sciences and/or patient care and is offered by an accredited post-secondary educational institution in the biologic sciences, physical sciences, radiologic sciences, health and medical sciences, social sciences, communication (verbal and written), mathematics, computers, management, or education methodology. Some subject areas that may NOT be applicable include courses in history, fine arts, geology, geography, and astronomy.

ARDMS: American Registry of Diagnostic Medical Sonographers

ASRT: American Society of Radiologic Technologists

Biennium: A period of time spanning two (2) years. As used in the ARRT renewal process, the start of the technologist's birthmonth every other year marks the beginning of a biennium. Because the ARRT's renewal process is linked to a technologist's birthmonth, the biennial period is likewise linked to the technologist's birthmonth.

Example 19.1: *A technologist with a January birthmonth would end one biennium on December 31, 1996, and begin a new biennium on January 1, 1997, which would continue through December 31, 1998.*

Example 19.2: *A technologist with a June birthmonth would end one biennium on May 31, 1997, and begin a new biennium on June 1, 1997, which would continue through May 31, 1999.*

CAMRT: Canadian Association of Medical Radiation Technologists

Category A Credit: An activity that qualifies as a Continuing Education Activity as defined in this document and which meets one of the following criteria, is awarded Category A credit.

---

1. Activities approved by one of the following RCEEMs:

American College of Radiology
American Healthcare Radiology
   Administrators
American Society of Radiologic
   Technologists
Canadian Association of Medical
   Radiation Technologists
Society of Diagnostic Medical
   Sonographers
Society of Nuclear Medicine -
   Technologists Section.
Society of Vascular Technology

2. Activities approved by one of the following other organizations:

American Medical Association -
   Category 1
American Nurses Association -
   ANCC

3. Academic Courses

4. CPR Certification through the Heart Association or the Red Cross

EXCEPTION Registrants who have completed CE requirements to maintain their license in the following states may designate the CE activities approved by their state licensing agency as Category A credit (see Section 14):

Florida	*Kentucky*
Iowa	*Oregon*
Illinois	*New Mexico*
Massachusetts	

Category B Credit: All Continuing Education Activities as defined in this document having not been approved for Category A credit.

Certification: The process of granting a certificate attesting to the demonstration of qualifications in a profession.

Example 19.3: A technologist receives a certificate after successfully passing an ARRT examination and meeting all other requirements for eligibility.

Contact Hour: Contact hour is defined as being equal to 50 to 60 minutes and is awarded one continuing education credit.

Continuing Education Activity: A learning activity that is planned, organized, and administered to enhance the professional knowledge and skills underlying professional performance that a technologist uses to provide services for patients, the public or the medical profession. In order to qualify as continuing education, the activity must be planned, organized and provide sufficient depth and scope of a subject area.

Continuing Education Credit: Unit of measurement for continuing education activities. One continuing education credit is awarded for one contact hour (50-60 minutes). Educational activities of 30-49 minutes of duration will be awarded one-half of one CE credit. Activities lasting less than 30 minutes will receive no credit.

CPR: Category A credit will be awarded for valid CPR certification. Credits are awarded on the date of the certification or re-certification. A copy of a valid certification card issued by the Red Cross or the Heart Association will serve as documentation. Only one of the following options will be allowed during a biennium:

(1.) CPR certification in Basic Life Support will automatically be awarded 3 Category A credits limited to 3 credits per biennium,
or
(2.) Advanced CPR certification (Advanced Life Support, Instructor, Instructor Trainer) will be awarded 6 Category A credits limited to 6 credits per biennium.

Documentation: Proof of participation in a particular educational activity. Documentation must include: name of participant, dates of attendance; title and content of the activity; number of contact hours for the activity; name of sponsor; signature of the instructor or an authorized representative of the sponsor issuing the documentation; and a reference number if the activity has been approved by a RCEEM.

Inservice Presentation: Inservice presentations that are general in content and would apply to a wide audience of technologists would be considered a CE activity. Inservice presentations that are an employment requirement or are specific to an institution will not be awarded CE credit.

Example 19.4: A course on universal precautions would be applicable for any technologist.

Example 19.5: A course on how the radiograph file folder is completed is specific to that facility and does not meet the definition of a CE activity.

NMTCB: Nuclear Medicine Technology Certification Board

Probation Status: Beginning in 1997, technologists who apply for renewal of registration of a certificate but who fail to meet the CE requirements will be placed on CE probation status. (See Section 11 of this document for more detailed information on probation status.)

Presentation: An educational activity in which the presenter prepares and orally presents a topic. With proper documentation, a presenter will receive 3 CE credits for the preparation of a presentation that has been evaluated and approved as a Category A activity, as well as 1 CE credit for each hour of actual presentation. This total must not exceed 12 credits per biennium.

Radiologic Technology: The health profession comprised of certified technologists who provide services for physicians, patients and the public. This "umbrella" term encompasses the imaging and therapeutic modalities in medical radiology.

Recognized Continuing Education Evaluation Mechanism (RCEEM): A mechanism for evaluating the content, quality, and integrity of an educational activity. The evaluation must include a review of educational objectives, content selection, faculty qualifications, and educational methods and materials. Among the requirements for qualification as a RCEEM, an organization must be national in scope, non-profit, radiology based, and must be willing to evaluate the CE activity developed by any technologist within a given discipline. The organization must demonstrate the need for an additional RCEEM and supply evidence of sufficient experience and resources to provide for the valid and reliable evaluation of CE activities.
Current organizations with RCEEM status include: ACR, AHRA, ASRT, CAMRT, SDMS, SNM-TS, and SVT.

Reinstatement: A technologist who fails to renew the registration of a certificate is no longer registered by the ARRT. In order to become registered again, the technologist must apply for reinstatement of the registration of the certificate and meet other requirements as set by the ARRT. (See Section 12 of this document.)

SDMS: Society of Diagnostic Medical Sonographers

SNM-TS: Society of Nuclear Medicine - Technologist Section

Sponsor: An organization responsible for the content, quality and integrity of the educational activity. A sponsor plans, organizes, supports, endorses, subsidizes and/or administers educational activities. (See Section 17 of this document.)

SVT: Society of Vascular Technology

Triennium: A period of time spanning three (3) years. As used in the ARRT renewal process, the triennium will only be assigned to currently registered technologists having a birth year ending in an odd number who have been certified prior to 1994. This triennium will begin on the first day of the technologist's birthmonth in 1995 and will end on the last day of the month preceding the technologist's birthmonth in 1998. The triennium will be used only at the initiation of the mandatory phase to stagger CE compliance periods of current registrants and only for registrants beginning the mandatory requirements in 1995.

Answers to Test Questions

Chapter 1

1. b
2. b
3. a
4. c
5. b
6. c
7. b
8. b
9. c
10. a
11. c
12. a = 3; b = 4; c = 1; d = 2
13. a = 1; b = 3; c = 4; d = 2; e = 5
14. e
15. a = 3; b = 1; c = 2; d = 5; e = 4

Chapter 2

1. a
2. e
3. d
4. d
5. a
6. d
7. e
8. a = 4; b = 3; c = 2; d = 1; e = 5
9. d
10. d

11. e
12. b
13. b
14. b
15. a

Chapter 3

1. e
2. a = 3; b = 2; c = 1
3. e
4. b
5. c
6. d
7. b
8. b
9. b
10. e
11. a
12. b
13. b
14. d
15. c
16. a
17. b
18. a
19. a
20. c
21. e

Chapter 4

1. b
2. a
3. b
4. b
5. d
6. a
7. d

8. c
9. e
10. b
11. e
12. a
13. a
14. e
15. b
16. e
17. a
18. a
19. c
20. b

Chapter 5

1. a
2. b
3. d
4. a
5. d
6. c
7. c
8. b
9. d
10. b
11. c
12. a
13. a
14. b
15. c
16. d
17. d
18. d
19. d
20. a

Chapter 6

1. e
2. a
3. b
4. e
5. a
6. b
7. d
8. b
9. c
10. a
11. e
12. e
13. c
14. a
15. a
16. e
17. a
18. a
19. c
20. b

Chapter 7

1. d
2. c
3. e
4. e
5. b
6. a
7. $a = 4; b = 3; c = 5; d = 4; e = 1$
8. e
9. e
10. $a = 2; b = 3; c = 5; d = 4; e = 1$
11. e
12. a
13. d
14. d
15. d

16. d
17. c
18. a
19. d
20. a
21. e
22. c
23. a
24. a
25. d

Chapter 8

1. d
2. d
3. d
4. c
5. e
6. e
7. d
8. d
9. b
10. c
11. c
12. e
13. e
14. a
15. b
16. a
17. b
18. b
19. b
20. b

Chapter 9

1. a
2. a
3. c

4. d
5. e
6. b
7. e
8. d
9. a
10. e
11. a
12. There is no specific right or wrong answer to this question.

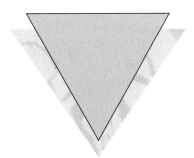

Index